Ageing, Disability and Spirituality

Ageing, Disability and Spirituality
Addressing the Challenge of Disability in Later Life

Edited by Elizabeth MacKinlay

Jessica Kingsley Publishers
London and Philadelphia

First published in 2008
by Jessica Kingsley Publishers
116 Pentonville Road
London N1 9JB, UK
and
400 Market Street, Suite 400
Philadelphia, PA 19106, USA

www.jkp.com

Library of Congress Cataloging in Publication Data
Ageing, disability, and spirituality : addressing the challenge of disability in later life / edited by Elizabeth MacKinlay.
    p. cm.
Includes bibliographical references.
ISBN 978-1-84310-584-8 (pb : alk. paper) 1. Older people--Religious life. 2. Church work with older people. 3. People with disabilities--Religious life. 4. Church work with people with disabilities. I. MacKinlay, Elizabeth, 1940- II. Title: Aging, disability, and spirituality.
BL625.4.A33 2008
362.6--dc22
                        2007035184
British Library Cataloguing in Publication Data
A CIP catalogue record for this book is available from the British Library

ISBN 978 1 84310 584 8

Printed and bound in Great Britain by
MGP Books Group, Cornwall

Contents

Acknowledgements

I acknowledge the commitment and contribution of each of the authors to the writing of this edited collection of essays. I am also pleased to acknowledge the valuable work of Karen Woodward in providing secretarial support and Merrie Hepworth for her valuable work of reading and checking the manuscript.

Preface

This collection of essays began with the preparation for the third national conference on ageing and spirituality, hosted by the Centre for Ageing and Pastoral Studies (CAPS). Each of the five conferences hosted by CAPS so far has focused on a different aspect of ageing and spirituality; this conference focused on disability. Disability in later life arises from two different perspectives: lifelong disabilities and acquired disabilities of ageing.

Authors of the major papers, selected concurrent presentations and workshops were invited to write on these important topics for this book. The perspective is a spiritual one, and the questions examined include: What does it mean to live with disabilities, mental and/or physical? What does it mean to be a person with disabilities? What does it mean to care for someone who has disabilities? How does spirituality assist people living with disabilities? What spiritual strengths can be drawn on by carers?

This is not a book that will tell you how to provide physical care for older people who have disabilities; there are other books that do that. This book focuses on the effects of the disabilities and how people may live effective and meaningful lives in the face of disability.

Aims of the conference were to bring researchers and practitioners together to share and examine issues of disability, spirituality and ageing, in the context of related theological and ethical issues. Emphasis was given to mental health disabilities common in later life, developmental disabilities and the psychosocial and spiritual effects on the person and their family. Emphasis was also given to issues faced by veterans in ageing and living with disabilities.

In recent years we have become much more aware of the issues surrounding mental health issues in later life. Dementia, in particular, and depression have gained higher focus and interest. But now, further challenges arise as ageing adult children with intellectual disabilities and their own ageing parents struggle with the patterns of a lifetime, seeking to adjust to ageing together.

The chapters of this book are arranged to present theological and ethical perspectives on the major themes of the book before introducing practice-related issues. The authors include academics and practitioners with backgrounds in theology, ethics, nursing, social work, psychology, diversional therapy and occupational therapy.

In Chapter 1, Elizabeth MacKinlay introduces the book with an overview of the issues of ageing, disability and spirituality that follow. The second chapter, by John Swinton, provides theological reflections on the concept of successful ageing, in the context of personhood and dementia. All that we do in working with older people who have disabilities is girded by ethics and Laurence McNamara presents a chapter where the motive of hospitality guides practice. MacKinlay's Chapter 4 considers emerging issues of disability in later life related not simply to the issues of acquired age-related disabilities, but also to the growing numbers of people living with lifelong disabilities, who are also ageing. The importance of pastoral response is highlighted. Eileen Glass takes up the theme of developmental disabilities as she writes of experiences of ageing both for people with intellectual disabilities and for their carers within L'Arche communities.

Christopher Newell challenges conceptions of disability as he asks questions around 'Better dead than disabled?' thus moving further into the debate over ethics and disability. Rosalie Hudson explores issues around dementia and ethics relating to care. The theme on ethics continues in Chapter 8, in which Lorna Hallahan looks particularly at the types of relationships people who are disabled have with those who are not.

Matthew Anstey brings a context of biblical reflection and scriptural reminiscence to disability in ageing. In Chapter 10, Malcolm Goldsmith reflects on the experiences and challenges of dementia in later life. The next chapter is jointly written by Christine Bryden and Elizabeth MacKinlay and is a continuation of Bryden's personal and spiritual journey into dementia. In the context of a multifaith and multicultural society, Ruwan Palapathwala presents a Buddhist perspective on pastoral care for people with disabilities. This perspective of focus on the people with disabilities is further illuminated by Dagmar Ceramidas as she examines the interplay of faith and depression in older age. Kirstin Robertson-Gillam describes a recent study of people with dementia and the use of choir work, while Carmen Moran explores humour and its links to meaning and spirituality among a number of veterans of the Second World War. Alan Niven provides an important chapter that offers a way of understanding the role of ritual in pastoral care.

CHAPTER 1

Introduction: Ageing, Disability and Spirituality

Elizabeth MacKinlay

It seems obvious that ageing and disability are associated. This is most readily seen in the physical changes and decrements of later life. The disabilities of ageing challenge the model of successful ageing proposed by Rowe and Kahn (1997), defined as 'low probability of disease and disease-related disability, high cognitive and physical functional capacity, and active engagement with life' (p.433). While this model is helpful to use in health promoting strategies for ageing, it sets those who live with disabilities outside the model. Critique of this model of ageing has included the concept of 'positive spirituality' (Crowther *et al.* 2002), the authors identifying 'positive' spirituality as the missing component of the model. Even adding positive spirituality to the model fails to produce an embracing holistic model for ageing. Successful ageing is essentially a wellness model of ageing and, as defined, isolates older people with disabilities, physical or mental, outside the model. Thus, viewed from outside the model of successful ageing, health for these people is often only to be considered in relation to medical treatments, not health promotion and well-being.

It is contended in this book that well-being is possible and achievable for many older people notwithstanding their disabilities. What is required is a willingness to look outside the disabilities, to see these people, not assessed according to various scales that would label them as being more or less worthy of care, but as persons, as much so as any other persons, with or without disability. Our responses to persons with disabilities are critical factors in the mix of complexities that surround the worth and value of people who have disabilities. These are the foci of this collection of essays based on issues of ageing, disability and spirituality.

11

Contexts of disability, ageing and spirituality

David Coulter, in his foreword to the collection of essays titled *Critical Reflections on Stanley Hauerwas' Theology of Disability* (Swinton 2004), notes that as a physician working with children having profound intellectual disabilities he came to realize that what he and they were sharing was their spirituality. That, he saw, 'did not depend on age, race, sex, wealth, or ability' (Swinton 2004, p.xv). Further, he wrote: 'Indeed [a "third look" is] to see in each other the ground of all being and existence, the transcendence or divinity that informs our spirituality' (p.xv). From this is drawn the concept of all persons being equal in human dignity, regardless of any disability; concluding that with this as the starting point, no one has to prove their worth as persons.

Reinders set out two perspectives on disabilities that he identified as attitudes towards people with disabilities. The first is 'Since you're here, we're going to care for you as best as we can.' The second is 'But everyone would be better off if you were not here at all' (Reinders 2000, p.4). He notes that although these messages are apparently separated, 'many people within the disability community are troubled by the relation between them' (p.4). Reinders' work in his 2000 publication is mostly concerned with disabilities at the beginning of life. In this book we examine disabilities at the later stages of life, in ageing, where perhaps even less value is afforded to those who are physically or, even more particularly, mentally disabled.

The topics in this book relating to ageing and disability mostly focus on dementia, depression, stroke, other mental health conditions, and developmental disabilities such as Down syndrome. At the base of these chapters lies the fundamental concept and understanding of people in relationship. Notions of individualism and autonomy are challenged as ways of being effective in society and community; on the other hand, interdependence is highlighted as a way of living that affirms the vulnerable as well as the strong.

Relationship, connectedness and disability

Nearly all of the issues discussed in this book revolve around relationship and connectedness in some way. Different authors have considered issues of relationship from different perspectives. For example, McNamara has used the notion of hospitality, with an idea of openness to the unexpected guest. This concept must recognize the centrality of friendship. He sees the gift of self to another in friendship as being of far more value than attaining autonomous existence. McNamara notes that friendship moves beyond ideas of ability or disability to 'enrich and enliven lives' (see Chapter 3, p.38).

Newell (Chapter 6) underlines the significance of relationship when he writes out of his own experiences of disability, asking whether it is 'better to be dead than disabled'. Apart from the obvious physical struggle Newell has encountered over many years of living with long-term disability, it is the lack of human compassion that seems to strike at him most severely. For him, his *being* as a person, a priest and disabled is central to his identity. He challenges the church and its attitudes towards and care for those who are disabled. One of his questions is how people who are disabled can minister to others. Further, he asks whether this is a legitimate role, or whether people with disabilities should be seen only in the role of disability that defines them. People with severe disabilities challenge those of us with the types of disabilities that we can hide from others. To take an alternative view, persons ought not to be defined by their disabilities; in situations where this occurs, we lose sight of the person, seeing only the disability. Healing and wholeness come as we are able, unselfconsciously, to connect with and accept other people, disabled or not, as our brothers and sisters. To live interdependently and in love, relating to the person not the disability, is the model advocated in Scripture and the work of Jesus. Real community is not simply about physical appearances, but about social, emotional and spiritual connectedness.

Hallahan (Chapter 8) also writes of the minimal participation of people with disabilities 'at the heart of congregational life'. She writes about the 'priority of belonging', noting that the differences are not primarily between people with disabilities and those without, but in the types of *relationships* people have (that are often based on the disability). The quality of the relationship may be primarily set by the perception the 'non-disabled' person has of a 'disabled' person. Hallahan notes that what is needed, in healing woundedness of those with disabilities, is reconciliation and relationship building. She writes of disabilities and spirituality, introducing a Celtic concept of the 'thin places', meaning a place of connecting with the 'holy other' or the deeper things of life. She sees these places as being where the marginalized live. We who care for others at critical times of their lives are privileged to be with them in these 'thin places'.

A theology of disability and ageing

Swinton (Chapter 2, p.25) points out that 'A key question thrown up by liberal society is whether the symptoms of dementia depersonalize the sufferer, that is, make them into non-persons'. Swinton chooses to take an alternative view of dementia and the people who have this condition. This is the view that affirms people because of who they *are*, not what they can *do*, based on the work of Kitwood (1997) that sees persons with dementia, not the disease first.

'The significance and personhood of the person with dementia is safeguarded and sustained within the very being of God quite apart from the relationships a person may or may not encounter at a temporal level' (p.31). This statement forms a linkage with a number of chapters in this book that look at what it means to be a person with a disability. Swinton makes an important point about the centrality of relationships for human beings. We have the ability to bestow personhood on others, simply through the manner of our relationships with them. We may affirm them, or we may reject them, labelling people with dementia as being 'non-persons'. Should we choose the latter view, then this will colour our relationships with and care of those with dementia. People who have dementia seem very able to detect attitudes of fear and rejection towards them.

Swinton includes the possibility of 'rementing' that can recover some lost capacities, in spite of cognitive loss. We have certainly found this to be possible in the long-term small group spiritual reminiscence research (MacKinlay and Trevitt 2006). Swinton takes Kitwood's construct one step further as he asks what the status is of the person who has no human relationships. His answer is a theological one, as he outlines the Trinitarian and divine relationship with those who have dementia. God remains with those who cannot cognitively remember. God's faithfulness does not desert the person with dementia; God-in-relationship remains. Swinton's perspective calls us to look beyond the diagnosis to the person within, who is always within the scope of God's love in Christ. 'We might forget God, but God will not and indeed cannot forget us… His remembering us when all seems to have been forgotten, is an inevitable outcome of his essential nature as Christ-for-us' (pp.31–2).

A perspective on ethics, ageing, disability and spirituality

Hauerwas presents an ethical perspective to the topic. He sees the secular position on mental disability as only providing hope for disabled people to the extent that they may be enabled to become independent. Hauerwas sets out an argument based on this being the wrong goal because 'We are creatures. Dependency, not autonomy, is one of the ontological characteristics of our lives' (2004a, p.16). This dependency is an essential factor that underlines the importance of human relationships. We need each other in community. Hauerwas notes the fact that we were created for each other and this has the effect of our being incomplete alone. The completeness of human beings comes through sharing of joy and suffering. When seen through Christian eyes, suffering cannot be seen as a reason to eliminate the person. This contrasts with the Western societal view of the primacy of autonomy. 'Christians are, or at least should be, imbedded in a narrative that makes possible a sharing of lives with one another that enables us to go on in the face of the inexplicable' (Hauerwas 2004a, p.16).

McNamara (in Chapter 3) gives emphasis to human bodiliness and our responses to each other as wounded healers, drawing on Nouwan's concept of the wounded healer. McNamara sets out the importance of our understanding of ourselves as embodied persons as we provide care, and work with older people who have disabilities. McNamara and other authors in this book challenge the liberal societal ethics stance. Thus we examine the nature of ageing, disability and spirituality within those who live these experiences, and we examine the nature of the providers of care and their effect on those they care for. Values of rationality, independence, and autonomous individuality lie against values of dependency, interdependency, and love. These ethical and theological perspectives are important starting points for this book and its overarching theme of ageing, disability and spirituality.

Further ethical perspectives are powerfully presented by Newell (in Chapter 6) as he struggles with his own ageing disabilities, being a priest and ministering within a church that seems to have at least some difficulties in accepting people with disabilities into holistic ministry of the church. This chapter could be termed a lament, as Newell honestly and openly shares his challenges within ministry and his experiences of disability and vulnerability within the church. Newell's chapter is set in a narrative of disability and life meaning. He suggests that a negative focus on disability results in missing the potentials for richness that can be found arising from living through the disabilities, even in the midst of pain.

Perceptions of dementia and the person

It is inevitable in a collection of papers such as these, on disability and ageing, that dementia will feature in the majority of papers. In the literature, a number of types of dementia are described; the most commonly occurring is Alzheimer's disease, the second most common is vascular dementia and third, Lewy body dementia (Woods 2005). It is also possible that more than one type of dementia can be present in the one person.

Two views of dementia currently dominate the literature. The first is the biomedical view of dementia as a disease of increasing cognitive decline that robs the person of abilities over a number of years, with increasing memory loss. The second view prefers to see dementia as more commonly associated with ageing, and questions that it is always a disease process. Woods (2005) states that it is increasingly clear from epidemiological studies where post-mortem examinations of brains of participants have been done that the dementia in those aged 75 years and older 'is less straightforward than the simple disease paradigm suggests' (p.252). He suggests numbers of questions still exist regarding dementia in advanced old age. Hughes, Louw and Sabat (2006) go further and state:

> At the most objective end of 'mental' illness...it turns out there is no hard scientific boundary between disease and normality. Lines can be drawn, but their exact location is a matter of evaluative judgement based on correlations between neuropathology and symptoms and signs. (p.2)

Hughes *et al.* then ask, 'Which symptoms and signs? How much forgetting is pathological? What counts as normal ageing?' But further emphasis needs to be given to finding a balanced model, pushing neither the biomedical model nor the moral model to the extreme or to the exclusion of the other. Further, what is needed is an holistic model of care that keeps the person at the centre. This model considers dementia in the context of physiological, psychological, social, spiritual, ethical and cultural dimensions. Hughes *et al.* (2006, p.4) contend that 'because of the ways in which dementia is thought of, the diagnosis itself amplifies any disabilities that may result from the pathology'. In a book that links disabilities, ageing and spirituality this statement is an important grounding for care of those with dementia, or indeed any type of later life disability. How easy it is to see only as far as the disability, and thus fail to see the person.

In Chapter 11, Christine Bryden writes as a wonderful advocate for people with dementia. She is an example of what is possible when people are able to openly dialogue about what it means to have dementia. She has been empowered to live life to the full, even in the presence of dementia. She has written out of her own experience of having dementia. She too writes of living with disability; in her struggle she finds that she is becoming more who she really is. Her faith has sustained her on a journey of 12 years now, from diagnosis of early onset Alzheimer's. Her courage is evident in the work she has done, reaching out to people in different parts of the world and bringing them hope for ways of living effectively with dementia. More recently she has become exhausted in the unrelenting pressures of speaking tours, and she feels that she cannot continue to speak publicly; her husband is doing much more of the speaking for her now.

Chapter 5, by Eileen Glass, provides a wonderful and moving account of living with people who are profoundly disabled. Eileen draws on her long experience of living in L'Arche communities and she demonstrates the central place of community and connectedness that make these communities so special. She writes: 'In many ways people with an intellectual disability represent the human heart unmasked and they can startle us with their directness, their transparency and their deep compassion' (p.59). Glass asks questions of the fundamental basis for our humanity. She asks challenging questions of each of us. What are the bases of our judgments? Or our prejudices? Although all of us have some disabilities, she notes that we are taught from an early age to hide and deny them. As other authors have noted, Glass also sees how those who have disabilities are ranked according to their capacities to measure up to societal standards. She notes further that we may become fearful that we too may be caught out and labelled because of our own hidden disabilities. In the L'Arche community, all people are valued, regardless of capacity or disability.

Fear as a barrier to well-being and to care

The topics of fear, ageing and disability are raised by several authors in this book. MacKinlay has written of fear leading to misunderstanding, and of that fear causing people to separate themselves from the person or object feared. Dementia is feared by many; it is not generally named or spoken about openly with people who have dementia, just as death is not often spoken about openly. Recently I was asked if it would be alright to tell other residents of an aged care facility that one of their friends in the facility had died. The question related to respecting the privacy of the person who had died. If fear drives the agenda, then compassion is driven out. The need of vulnerable elderly people to know about their friends must be honoured. To deny the reality of life and death on the basis of 'privacy' is to move outside any compassionate understanding within society. It is a common human tendency to fear things that are outside our experience; but there is something more required of us, and that is to move beyond our personal fear, the fear that binds us and prevents us being able to reach out in love to others. Both Goldsmith and Glass address these issues.

A model of spiritual tasks and process of ageing is the basis for MacKinlay's response to people with disabilities. This model examines disability and ageing through people's needs for connectedness, search for meaning in the face of disability, of finding identity through story, through use of symbols and ritual. Hope is made possible through finding one's true identity, being able to transcend seemingly insurmountable challenges, and rest in the strength that may be present in God or other deities.

Time and dementia

In the workplace time may be a powerful force, requiring the meeting of deadlines and the reaching of certain specified outcomes by pre-ordained dates and times. Outside of a work environment however, time takes on different meaning. Is it really important that we know what day it is? Much of our knowledge and sense of time is contextual. It is one thing to say that time goes too quickly; it is another to know what today is – is it Friday? Does it matter? In dementia, and maybe even on holidays, labelling of time becomes less urgent, and the need may disappear altogether.

Bryden, as her dementia progresses, talks of living in the present moment; it is all that seems to make sense to her now; the future is unknown, the past cannot be remembered with any certainty, or not at all. This time surely is God's time, not chronological time, perhaps 'the eternal now' of Paul Tillich, as written of by Mel Kimble in discovering time in a new way following his diagnosis of cancer – 'With a greater awareness of my finitude and mortality, time and its passing took on deeper meaning. I was learning and experiencing the difference between *chronos*, calendar time, and *kairos*, eschatological time that involves my ultimate destiny' (Kimble 2001, p.152). Perhaps there are connections between what Bryden and Kimble were experiencing, one because of cognitive decline (and increased awareness of her mortality) and the other because of the diagnosis of cancer. Bryden also noted (2005) that living in the present is a new experience, with a letting-go of the anxieties that surround the making and keeping of priorities. This new way of being is a resting in God's presence, eternally in the present.

On the other hand, Goldsmith suggests 'there are different times, different phases that people with dementia and their carers pass through, each possessing the possibilities for growth and nourishment whilst also containing the seeds of possible despair and dissolution' (Chapter 10, p.122). The sense of time is perhaps seen differently by those who wait and care when contrasted with those who have dementia. Questions of time arise for those who care: 'How long?' Goldsmith writes of dementia as being a time of waiting through the long progress of the disease and adopting attitudes that watch for and appreciate the sacrament of the present moment. This time also involves mystery and suffering.

Power and disempowerment

McNamara notes that too often relationships are understood in terms of power and violence (see Chapter 3, p.36). It is too easy to disempower people who have disabilities. One of the ways that people are disempowered is through the process of labelling. Labelling – mentally disabled, mentally handicapped, Down syndrome, dementia, Alzheimer's – places a person in a category of expected behaviours and capacities together with the expected and socially sanctioned repertoire of ways of responding and reacting to them. Hauerwas (2004a, p.19) notes that the only benefits of the process of labelling may be to 'the agents of intervention'. Further, Hauerwas writes, the issue 'is not just the label, but who gets to use the label' (2004b, p.196). Issues of power are thus intricately bound up in labelling.

Hudson, in Chapter 7, emphasises differences between societal values that promote individualism and Christian values that affirm community. Backing this is her discussion on the language used to describe dementia and those who have dementia; the language chosen can serve to separate those who have dementia from those who do not, as people with dementia become labelled. Hudson suggests that use of language can either enable or disable persons, and the power of language may be at the base of separation of these vulnerable people from others in community. Hudson illustrates how it is possible either to increase the disability experienced by people who have disabilities, or to enable their well-being through our attitudes and approaches to them.

Ways of meeting the challenges and supporting, affirming, and honouring older people who live with disabilities, and relate to spirituality, well-being and pastoral care, are discussed in the remaining chapters.

Anstey, in Chapter 9, examines the concept of scriptural reminiscence in relationship to narrative gerontology. This unusual approach to ageing and reminiscence is taken by a scholar of Hebrew who makes connections between Scripture and the ageing process. Narrative is being more widely used in gerontology as a means of life review, reconciliation and completion of the life story (Kenyon, Clark and de Vries 2001). In this collection of essays, Anstey explores the application of narrative for older and disabled people, through engagement with scriptural reminiscence. This provides a way of connecting the life journey of the individual and the faith community with the collective journey of faith recorded in Scripture. It is a practical means of affirming the worth and value of older people and assisting them towards further growth in their spiritual lives. This becomes a means of recognizing personal identity, and in this case, the story of Jacob is presented as a way into disability and the faith story.

A multicultural and multifaith perspective on ageing, disability and pastoral care is brought by Palapathwala in Chapter 12 on Buddhist perspectives of disability in ageing as he considers pastoral care in a Buddhist context.

Robertson-Gillam, in Chapter 14, reports on a study done in a residential aged care facility, using choir work with people who have dementia and are depressed. This was a valuable pilot study, clearly demonstrating the potential benefits of using music in the setting of a choir. There is no doubt that this was of great value to those engaged in the choir work.

Humour and spirituality in ageing

Moran (Chapter 15) explored the use of humour by older veterans in reminiscences of their time at war in the Second World War. She found less use of humour than she had expected; however, she did find instances of the spiritual dimension in her study. Moran found that many of the older veterans had talked very little or not at all about their war experiences. Some were only beginning to speak of these times 60 years later, perhaps in the context of reminiscence. For some the trauma of these earlier events in their young and impressionable lives was still to be resolved. These realizations may be important in pastoral care for this group of older veterans.

Depression and the faith journey

Ceramidas reports in Chapter 13 on some aspects of her doctoral study into the relationship between depression and Christian faith in later life. Depression is yet another disability that leads to reduced quality of life for older people. Ceramidas' work has shown a relationship between people's perceived closeness of relationship with God and how well they were able to cope with episodes of depression.

Ageing, disability and ritual

Niven has made the connections between the experiences of the life journey and relationship, both human and divine, in Chapter 16, which explores the place of ritual in ageing and disability. This is an important chapter, weaving connections between a theology of ritual, ourselves as carers, the persons in need of ritual and the relationship of equality in the process of participation in effective ritual.

Conclusion

There is much to examine in these issues of ageing, disability and spirituality. Ageing is more than 'successful' ageing; it is about living life to the full regardless of disabilities. Further, life is about interdependence, rather than the autonomy espoused by the successful ageing movement. The context of these topics on disability is important. First, how are older people who are also disabled thought about? Attitudes towards and about people with disabilities will set the stage for relationships with them, or even the desire not to have relationships with them. Challenges include realizing that we, who may or may not be less disabled than those we work with and care for, still have a great deal that we can learn about being human from those with disabilities.

In the chapters ahead, the theology of disability and ageing is considered, and issues of ethical living and disabilities and of perceptions of dementia and the person are examined. Barriers to well-being, such as fear, the misuse of power and the possibility of disempowerment, are engaged with. The book concludes with several chapters on working with elderly people, using choir work, scriptural reminiscence and multifaith perspectives of ageing and pastoral care. The chapter on ritual challenges carers to become more aware of their own everyday rituals and examine ways of honouring rituals, especially at critical life points.

CHAPTER 2

Remembering the Person: Theological Reflections on God, Personhood and Dementia

John Swinton

Dementia is a difficult and painful condition. It is difficult and painful not simply because of the biological consequences of the deterioration of the brain and the relational consequences that this initiates, but also because experiencing such deterioration within a society which is deeply liberal in its political and philosophical assumptions means that dementia is necessarily perceived in deeply negative terms. The liberal worldview venerates a specific set of capacities, values, assumptions and expectations: the primacy of reason, rationality, cognitive ability, independence and the capacity for self-advocacy. Not only are these capacities deemed necessary for entry into the socio-political system, for example through the various social contracts that make up the matrix of society, they are also perceived as vital dimensions of what it means to be a person and to live in a manner which can truly be called human. The loss of intellectual functions such as thinking, remembering, and reasoning takes on a particularly negative set of meanings within liberal culture. Personhood is defined precisely by those aspects of experience that people with dementia lose as their condition progresses. From the outset then it is important to recognize that dementia is a cultural as well as a biomedical illness.

In this chapter I want to explore some aspects of this complex cultural milieu and how it impacts upon the ways in which people with dementia are perceived, understood and treated. In so doing I will challenge conventional understandings of personhood and begin to develop a theological perspective which will preserve the fullness of the personhood of people with dementia in all circumstances, and open up the possibility of developing forms of caring practices which move beyond culturally constructed assumptions and towards the person with dementia as a person with hope and possibilities. I will begin with a story: my story.

A narrative of sadness

I remember the first time I walked on to a 'dementia ward' some 30 years ago. I was 17 and it was the first day of my psychiatric nurse training. I had no idea what was going to happen. The only thing I was certain about was that I did not want to be there. The place was noisy and it stank of urine and faeces. 'Bodies' were wandering all around me; strange, lost souls with no apparent goal, just wandering; sometimes whispering to themselves, sometimes shouting to others who seemed to remind them of something or someone hidden deep within their past. I felt as though I was drowning in a terrifying sea of babbling, dishevelled, 'crazy' people. I had never been on a ward before – any ward, never mind this! This was an initiation of fire. At first I sought solace in the television room. Perhaps if I sat very quietly and watched television they would leave me alone and I could finish up my shift and slip home before they noticed I was gone! But it was not to be. I had only been there for ten minutes when the charge nurse ordered me to go and change an elderly man who had been incontinent. So, I and a nursing assistant took this gentleman into the open, public toilet to change him. As we wrestled with him to get his trousers off, the smell of faeces almost overpowering us, other patients wandered past, staring blankly at us as if we were not really there. It was like a scene from Bedlam.

And that day set the pattern for the rest of my time in that ward: a daily round of routine wherein warehoused 'non-persons' were given the basics of care within a context which seemed to assume that, whoever these people might have been, they were no longer worthy of more than basic care and minimal respect. And yet, as I began to get to know Chrissie and Charlie and Derek and all the other persons who lived out their final days within that hope-less context, I began to see things differently. I began to realize that these people were not 'lost souls', they were people; people with long and fascinating histories who had contributed greatly to the world. Certainly they had lost a lot. In a real sense they had forgotten who and whose they were. Yet there was much that they still retained. They still laughed and cried, they still enjoyed the warmth of human contact, they were still, if you were prepared to listen and take the time to engage, easily recognizable as valuable people with unique personalities. They still told stories; these often made no sense within their present context, but they provided echoes and resonances of lives lived well. The longer I worked with people whose life experience included dementia, the more I realized that the act of forgetting may not be the sole domain of the dementia sufferer. It seemed to me more that it was the system and, sometimes, those of us who sought to offer care within that system, who frequently 'forgot' people's status as unique persons created to be in meaningful loving relationships with others and with God.

Moving on?

Some twenty years later I found myself returning to that same ward, in a new role as a hospital chaplain. Much had changed. The attitudes and routines were considerably less rigid, more compassionate and thoughtful. At one level the system appeared to be beginning to see people with dementia as significant persons in need of care, love, recognition and sometimes protection. And yet, as I began to spend time with people with dementia and talk to carers, it was clear that the ways in which services were set up, the lack of time that professional carers had to spend with people, the shortage of staff and the general expectation of the institution meant that it was still very easy to 'forget' the personhood of people experiencing dementia. Some of the structures had certainly changed and some of the practices carried out by individuals were excellent, but the subtle shadow of warehousing and the not so subtle demands of caring for profit raised the awkward question of precisely what kind of commodity people with dementia were assumed to be. Why is it that we seem to struggle to remember and hold on to the personhood of people with dementia and to provide models of care and support that reflect this?

The biology of dementia

When narrated from the perspective of biomedicine dementia is inevitably perceived primarily as a narrative of pathology and loss. It is defined as a clinical state which is characterized by a catastrophic loss of function in multiple cognitive domains.

> Diagnostic features include: memory impairment and at least one of the following: aphasia, apraxia, agnosia, disturbances in executive functioning. In addition, the cognitive impairments must be severe enough to cause impairment in social and occupational functioning. Importantly, the decline must represent a decline from a previously higher level of functioning. (French 1995)

And of course dementia is indeed a narrative of profound loss both for sufferers and for those who care for them. This cannot and must not be underplayed. The question is: is this the *only* story that can be told about the lives of people with dementia?

Dementia and personhood

We have already looked at the way in which cultural assumptions relating to the criteria for meaningful personhood can be highly problematic for people with dementia. A key question thrown up by liberal society is whether the symptoms of dementia depersonalize the sufferer, that is, make them into non-persons. A good example of the consequences of such debate is found in the work of the Australian ethicist Peter Singer. Singer argues, from liberal presuppositions, that the central tenets of personhood reside in the human ability for 'self-awareness, self-control, a sense of the future, a sense of the past, the capacity to relate to others, concern for others, communication and curiosity' (Singer 1993, p.86). For current purposes it will be helpful to draw attention to two aspects of Singer's definition:

1. its liberal assumptions

2. its emphasis on *function* as definitive of personhood.

According to this understanding, human beings do not find their worth in what they are in and of themselves, but rather by what they are capable of *doing*, or what they *do not* or *cannot* do. The essence of personhood resides in and is determined by such human functions as memory, reason, self-consciousness, autonomy and self-advocacy. It is not enough for someone simply to be human. To be a person one needs to be able to have particular capacities and to carry out specific functions without which the morally protective label of 'person' cannot be ascribed.

Of course, the attributes highlighted by Singer are precisely the attributes which the condition of dementia takes away from the sufferer. This leads to Singer being able to advocate and argue strongly for the involuntary killing of people with dementia on the grounds that they are no longer persons (Singer 1993, p.192). This leaves us with the rather odd situation wherein human beings can be persons for 60, 70, 80 years, and live under the protection of this particular notion of personhood, only to find themselves living out their final years as non-persons who suddenly (or gradually) become less worthy of moral attention and protection. This offers a bleak future for a large section of the population who will inevitably encounter dementia and in so doing lose their status as persons. Such discussions place people with dementia in a very tenuous position. As Stanley Rudman puts it, 'It is clear that the emphasis on rationality easily leads to diminished concern for certain human beings such as infants... and the senile, groups of people who have, under the influence of both Christian and humanistic considerations, been given special consideration' (Rudman 1997, p.49). But of course, the person is not lost to dementia. If we look a little closer, another much more positive story begins to emerge.

Re-thinking dementia: from 'inevitable pathology' to person-in-relation

In developing an alternative narrative, it will be helpful to examine the work of the English psychologist Tom Kitwood. Whilst acknowledging the very real loss that people with dementia encounter, Kitwood presents an important counter-argument, suggesting that dementia should be reframed in terms of what people with dementia *are* and *can* do rather than what they are not and cannot do. Central to Kitwood's position is the suggestion that while dementia may be organic in origin, the actual life experiences of people living with this condition are not as determined by fading neurological activity as is commonly assumed.

He argues that our understanding of dementia has been constructed by a cluster of discourses, of which the dominant one is grounded in medical science (Kitwood 1995). Within this interpretative framework, the person is totally subsumed to their neurological condition, even to the point where, linguistically, they are frequently referred to as 'dead'. The possibility that the person may remain, despite the ravages of their condition, is often not even considered. The reason for this, Kitwood suggests, is that dementia has become so medicalized that other ways of interpreting and understanding the person's condition are almost totally subsumed to the power of the medical interpretation.

> Throughout the many debates on the causes and treatments of senile dementia and indeed in much of the literature on dementia care, certain questions are very rarely asked. Who is the dementia sufferer? What is the experience of dementing really like? How can those who have a dementing illness be enabled to remain persons in the full sense? That they are experiencing subjects, with cognitions, intentions, desires, emotions, there can be no doubt. In the dominant discourse, however, and in some of the subordinate discourses also, dementia sufferers are present largely as an absence. Those who are recognizable as persons are the carers. The dementia sufferers themselves are not; rather, they are defined out of the world of persons, even to the extent of it being claimed, almost literally, that those in the later stages are already dead. (Kitwood 1995, p.153)

Whilst not using the same conceptual language, Kitwood here indicates the tensions between the natural and the social history of dementia and the negative consequences that occur when either one is given priority over the other. Due to the power of the medical interpretation of dementia (the natural history), the *person* behind the diagnostic label (their social history) has been 'lost' from the debate about what dementia is, and what constitutes effective dementia care (Swinton 2000a).

Returning to the question of personhood

Kitwood offers an alternative definition of personhood which challenges functional understandings in important ways. He defines personhood not in terms of functionality, but in terms of relationship: '[personhood] is a standing or status that is bestowed upon one human being by others, in the context of relationships and social being. It implies recognition, respect and trust' (Kitwood 1997, p.8). In this understanding, personhood is not a personal attribute that is dependent on capabilities or function. Personhood is the product of a particular form of relational encounter. To be a person requires one to be in a particular type of relationship with another person who is willing to bestow one with recognition, respect and trust. Personhood is not an individual achievement. It is a gift of community. Rather than conceiving of human beings as isolated, individual monads who in a sense both create and own their personhood, in Kitwood's perspective, community comes first; individuals emerge from and are shaped by the types of relationships that occur as they participate in some form of community.

Something more?

Kitwood also understands the development of the brain in a way that is helpful for current purposes. He argues that the growth of the brain is epigenetic rather than fixed and linear. He hypothesizes that the brain functions on three levels (Kitwood 1997, p.151). At the first level we have the structural condition of the brain that is established over the lifetime of the individual. This level of brain functioning is open to the rigours of time and disease processes, and is inevitably deteriorating throughout a person's life. It is degeneration within the physical structure of the brain that causes the process of dementing.

The second level is hypothetical. 'It is the highest level of mental functioning that is possible when a person's brain is in a particular structural state…the upper limits to mental functioning are set by the structural state of the brain' (p.151).

The third level comprizes the actual mental functioning of the person. Kitwood points out that the actual functioning of all people is considerably lower than their potential functioning. None of us ever achieves maximum brain function. Consequently the human brain has a depth of reserve functioning that is rarely if ever used.

If Kitwood's hypothesis is correct, there is no necessary correlation between level one and level three. We cannot realistically hope to understand and define dementia simply by exploring level one (i.e. the purely biological level). Indeed, to attempt to do so is a serious error which can have significant negative impact on people experiencing dementia. However, as Kitwood points out, 'this error is made repeatedly, and the findings of medical science are called in as a testimony to its truth' (p.152).

Secondly, and importantly for current purposes, if we accept that there may well be regions of the person's brain that remain undeveloped despite the ravages of dementia, this opens up space to explore ways in which the person's brain functioning may be enhanced or diminished through non-neurological interventions such as the provision of particular types of relationships, contexts and environments within which a person's spiritual and relational needs are prioritized (p.152).

Such a suggestion is not without a degree of empirical foundation. There is some evidence to suggest that given an appropriate social, relational and spiritual environment, a degree of *rementing* can take place in people with dementia. In particular, Sixmith and colleagues (Sixsmith, Stilwell and Copeland 1993) in a study of 'homely homes' where the care was of a very high quality found

> clear examples of 'rementing', or measurable recovery of powers that had apparently been lost; a degree of cognitive decline often ensued, but it was far slower than that which had been typically expected when people with dementia are in long term care. (Kitwood 1997, p.62)

It is for these reasons that Kitwood makes a strong plea for a movement away from the medicalization of dementia towards a model which takes seriously the wholeness and inherent relationality of persons and the significance of the natural interconnectivity of body, mind and soul for recovery and quality of life. This perspective moves us away from approaches to personhood that are based primarily on autonomy, self-determination and cognitive capacities, towards a perspective which offers a strong place for the significance of relationships, emotions, feelings and non-cognitive experiences.

A theology of dementia care

Important as Kitwood's position is for current purposes, it is not without its problems, primary amongst them being the lack of the transcendent in his understanding of relationality. If personhood is determined by human relationships-in-community alone, what happens to those who do not have access to such meaningful personal relationships? What happens to those whom others refuse to recognize as persons and who are deprived of the opportunity to attain meaningful personal relationships (the outcast, the lonely, the forgotten, the hermit, those who have forgotten who they are relating to)? Do they cease to be persons? In order to grasp the significance of Kitwood's perspective and its significance for specifically Christian care of people with dementia, we need to introduce a theological element which, whilst taking seriously the significance of human relationships, reaches beyond their limitations and anchors personhood in that which is in, yet beyond, human relationships and community.

God, Trinity and human relationality

Elsewhere I have argued for a relational conception of the human being based on Trinitarian theology (Swinton 2000b). There I made a case for human relationality to be viewed as analogous with Divine relationality; the inherently relational nature of human beings emerges from the nature and relational shape of the God in whose image they are created; a Trinitarian God who is Himself constituted by relationships. In this understanding God, understood as a Divine Trinity, is defined in social terms, as a perichoretic community of love; God the Father, God the Son and God the Holy Spirit, inextricably interlinked in an eternal community of loving relationship (Moltmann 1985, 1993). The concept of perichoresis indicates both distinction and complete unity or communion; a co-existence of each member with the other. Such a conception of God as Trinity suggests a divine, transcendent society or community of three fully personal and fully divine individuals, unified by their common divinity, that is, by the possession by each of the whole divine essence. Within such a context love is directed towards human beings, but primarily and archetypically towards the other persons of the Trinity. God is therefore 'He who has His being in personal, loving, dynamic relations of communion' (Feenstra and Plantinga 1989, p.27). Within such a conception of God, the creation of humanity – whose inherent relationality is a direct product of being made in the image of this Trinitarian God – is understood as the product of the overspill of this divine perichoretic love. Thus it can be seen that human beings are created *from* and *in* loving relationships, *for* loving relationships. Love *is* the essence of God's nature; God is love (1 John 4:8). The relational nature of human personhood is thus seen to be analogous to Divine personhood.

A Christological perspective

Here I would like to build on this basic understanding by adding an important Christological perspective which is vital for understanding both the way in which God remains with us and for us even when we can no longer cognitively be with and for God, and how those who follow the Trinitarian God who is love can understand themselves in relation to people with dementia. In order to achieve this, I will draw on the thinking of the German theologian Dietrich Bonhoeffer. A contextual reflection on Bonhoeffer's Christology as it can be used to relate to the experiences of people with dementia will provide a vital theological foundation for dementia care. Central to the argument that will be developed here is the suggestion that God remains with us and for us even when we cannot grasp the significance of that relationship with our cognitive senses. If God is with and for the person with dementia, then those who claim to follow God are called to be with and for the person with dementia in quite particular ways.

God with us and for us

In his Christology lectures Bonhoeffer offers a challenging perspective on the nature of Christ and the type of relationship that God offers to human beings. He suggests that

> Christ is Christ not as Christ in himself, but in relation to me. His being Christ is his being *pro me*. This being *pro me* is in turn not meant to be understood as an effect which emanates from him, or as an accident; it is meant to be understood as the essence, as the being of the person himself. This personal nucleus itself is the *pro me*. That Christ is *pro me* is not an historical or ontical statement, but an ontological one. That is, Christ can never be thought of in his being in himself, but only in his relationship to me. That in turn means that Christ can only be conceived of existentially, viz. in the community... It is not only useless to meditate on a Christ in himself, but even Godless. (Bonhoeffer 1978, pp.47–8)

This passage sums up something of the essence of Bonhoeffer's Christology. If we are to understand Christ we must understand the relationship of Christ to human beings; the very being of Christ is his being-for-humanity. More, it is impossible to reflect on Christ-in-Christ's-self without reflecting on his relationships to humanity. In Christ God creates a space within God's self for human beings; God opens up God's very being to incorporate human beings in such a way that it is not possible to understand Christ without recognizing his relatedness to and desire to relate to human beings. 'Christ can be thought of only in relational terms. "Being-there-with-and-for-us" is the manner of his existence and presence... Christ exists "as community"' (Bonhoeffer 1978, p.216). Indeed, in Bonhoeffer's perspective, to reflect on Christ without reflecting on his relatedness to human beings is a Godless act. This relatedness is not theoretical; nor does it relate only to the historical Jesus. Christ's relatedness to human beings is active and contemporary. God is *pro me* in the present as well as in the past. 'The humanity is taken up into the Trinity not since eternity, but from now to all eternity.' God is with us and for us now in a way that is unchangeable. Christ *is* the one who is for others; his sociality towards and for human beings is ontological. As Jenson puts it, 'This new thing of and in God (that it is new is clear from the fact that this is "from *now* to eternity" is an extension of God's identity to include humanity' (Jenson in John de Grucy (ed.) 1996, p.152).

Bonhoeffer views the human self as analogous to this inherent relatedness of Christ (Bonhoeffer 1998). The human self is inherently social, formed in self/other relationships. In like manner to the suggestion that Christ can only be understood as Christ-in-community, so also human beings can only be understood as they relate with one another and with God. The human person is created to be with and for others and with God in a way that is analogous to the way in which Christ is with and for human beings.

Creating space for the other

This Christological perspective has an important implication for the ways in which we frame the care of people with dementia. If in Christ God has opened up his very being in relationship to human beings, there is nothing that can change that. God remains with and for the person with dementia even when the person can no longer be with and for God, at least not in a cognitive sense. The significance and personhood of the person with dementia is safeguarded and sustained within the very being of God quite apart from the relationships a person may or may not encounter at a temporal level. We might forget God, but God will not and indeed cannot forget us. When we can no longer minister to God and to others, the God who is with us and for us will minister to us in our hour of need. God's coming to us in our weakness, His remembering us when all seems to have been forgotten, is an inevitable outcome of his essential nature as

Christ-for-us. Christ's *pro me*, his unending friendship, carries us and sustains our personhood even when we can no longer minister to him.

Mary's story

A story will help to contextualize these points. Margaret Hutchison, a nurse, tells the following story of her experience with a woman who has developing dementia.

An elderly lady suffering from dementia, paced the corridors of the nursing home restlessly – repeating over and over, just one word. The staff were disconcerted, but no one seemed quite sure how to calm her and put her mind at rest. In fact they were at a loss to understand the reason for her distress. The word she repeated over and over again was God – and that was all she said. One day a nurse got alongside her and walked with her up and down the corridors until eventually in a flash of inspiration she asked the lady, 'Are you afraid that you will forget God?' 'Yes, Yes!' she replied emphatically. The nurse was then able to say to her, 'You know even if you should forget God, He will not forget you. He has promised that.' For this lady who was forgetting many things, and was aware of it, that assurance was what she needed to hear. She immediately became more peaceful, and that particular behaviour ceased. She was responding positively to care which extended beyond the needs of body and mind – care of the human spirit. (Hutchison 1997)

This woman's revelation about the sustaining love of God which reaches beyond memory and the ability to reciprocate cognitively is crucial. Human beings are indeed persons-in-relation. Who we become is in a very real sense profoundly shaped by those whom we encounter. But ultimately our identity as persons and our hopes and possibilities for the future are determined and sustained by God who in Christ, is with us and for us even, and perhaps particularly in our darkest hours of need.

Conclusion: personhood as an act of faith

God looks through the tangles and confusions to our hearts to see what He Himself wrote there, Jesus Christ.[1]

This chapter has offered an argument for the personhood of people with dementia to be perceived as real and ever-present even in the midst of the experience of severe dementia. Kitwood's hypothesis on the epigenetic development of the brain suggests that we simply do not and cannot know the cognitive level that people are working at, or indeed have the potential to function at. Whilst their outer appearance may well reflect chaos and loss, there may well be hidden depths to a person's experience which, if the key can only be found, may reveal new and healing perspectives on their situation. Thus whilst a person's situation may appear to be hopeless, in reality there always remains the possibility of 'something more'.

None of this is intended to minimize the very real pain experienced by people whose loved ones face the outworking of this condition. While we may not want to argue that personhood is lost to the illness, there is no question that often the person-as-we-once-knew-them encounters radical changes. Iozzio, reflecting on her own family's experiences with her father, who had Alzheimer's disease, captures something of the deep loss that accompanies dementia for all concerned:

> Lovers, once intimately attuned to each other's rhythms, find themselves negotiating life's blessings and curses with a stranger. Children, having managed adult relationships with their parents, find themselves in reversed roles mothering or fathering them. Sisters and brothers, after fiercely asserting their uniqueness, find themselves holding desperately to the old familiar. Not suspecting the moment when I am no longer recognizable to my lover, parent, brother, friend, I am caught off guard by their unknowing. How do I remain faithful to them when they question, because of my Alzheimer's dementia, who I am? (Iozzio 2005, p.51)

To retain a sense that the person before us is fully a person when such profound changes are occurring is not an easy task for the carer, be they professional or lay. To recognize people as fully human when they have forgotten who they are, who you are and to whom they ultimately belong, requires more than psychological reframing; it requires an act of faith. The writer to the Hebrews describes faith thus: 'Faith is being sure of what we hope for and certain of what we do not see' (Hebrews 11:1). In order for us to hold on to the personhood and the full humanity of someone who appears to have been stripped of both, we need to be sure of what we hope for and certain of what we do not see. We need to develop a faith that is based on the theological certainties highlighted in this chapter and supported by the types of philosophical and psychological insights which assure us that our faith is not in vain. When this happens, Christians can begin to construct a different story around the experience of dementia and begin their task of caring at a different place; a place where it is not assumed that the story of dementia is nothing but a natural history of loss and devastation, but is rather a narrative of a fragmented human person who is held and sustained in their uniqueness by a God who has promised never to abandon them (Romans 8:39); a unique individual who requires the offer (but not the imposition) of relationships that can affirm them in their personhood and in their relationship with God. This theological dynamic allows us in faith to grasp (sometimes with great difficulty) the truth that the person before us may have changed in quite profound ways, but that they nonetheless remain persons loved by God and in need of friendship and love. Such a position is the foundation of Christian care.

As, in faith, the person experiencing dementia is held and sustained within the affirming boundaries of human and divine relationships, they are *re-membered*. To re-member something is to bring back together that which has been fragmented. To re-member a person with dementia is to offer them the kind of relational environment which mirrors God's loving, remembrance and unchanging embrace and, in so doing, draws back together the wholeness of the person whose life has been fragmented by the experience of dementia. Such a relationship both *re-members* the person and *remembers* for them. As Iozzio puts it:

> As long as my father lives, the work of my brothers/my aunts and uncles, my cousins, my husband and me is to *remember* for him. We work to put him back together, to *re-place* him in our relationships, to *remember* his sense of self. Even as he continues to lose his sense of self, which has been bound up in relationality to my mother and our family these many years, we are to remind him of his place among and with us. Even as the dementia of [Alzheimer's disease] causes him to not know us we are to know him. And even as he barely resembles the man he used to be – commanding, decisive, large – he is still husband, father, brother-in-law, and uncle to us. Fidelity asks this much of us, that we remain with him even as he fails to remember us, abandonment is not an option. (Iozzio 2005, p.64)

What can be said of fidelity can also be said of faith: *abandonment is not an option*.

In closing we will do well to remember the words of Jesus to the criminal on the cross who shouted: 'Jesus, remember me when you begin ruling as king!' Then Jesus said to him, 'Listen! What I say is true: Today you will be with me in Paradise!' (Luke 23:42–43). The truth of these words is the source of our hope and our joy. We will not be forgotten.

Notes

This chapter is published in an extended form as 'Forgetting Whose We Are: Theological Reflections on Personhood, Faith and Dementia' in the *Journal of Religion, Disability and Health*, 11, 1, pp.37–63 (2007). It is published here with the permission of The Haworth Press: Copyright © 2006, The Haworth Press, Inc., Binghamton, NY.

1   I am grateful to my friend and colleague Donald Meston, assistant chaplain at Aberdeen's Cornhill Hospital, for this quotation. The original source is unknown.

CHAPTER 3

Ethics, Ageing and Disability

Laurence McNamara

Introduction

For many years I have pondered Henri Nouwen's understanding of the 'wounded healer'. With him I have asked how wounds can become the source of healing (Nouwen 1972). Answering this question takes us into the mystery of Christian discipleship and how it engages the strengths and limits of our creaturely existence in the world. For Nouwen care of others demands the virtue of hospitality. Such hospitality has a healing power for, on the one hand, it necessitates that the host feel at home in their own house and, on the other, it creates a free and fearless place for the unexpected visitor. This calls to mind Jesus' visit to the home of Martha and Mary. It was Mary's single-minded attention to her guest that the Lord commended. Hospitality such as that of Mary in the gospels transcends the individual, for, to quote Nouwen,

> hospitality becomes community as it creates a unity based on the shared confession of our basic brokenness and on a shared hope. This hope in turn leads us far beyond the boundaries of human togetherness to Him who calls His people away from the land of slavery to the land of freedom. (Nouwen 1972, p.95)

This notion of hospitality provides a useful framework to discuss the topic of ethics, ageing and disability. Too often in today's world relationships are understood in terms of power or even violence. Some have even gone so far as to argue that all we can expect in contemporary societies is an ethic suitable for 'moral strangers' (Engelhardt 1986). The increasing polarization between the West and Islam also indicates that religion, political ideology, and the role of reason in the human enterprise will progressively influence our thinking in the decades ahead.

In this chapter I propose to develop three perspectives. In the first section I shall briefly explore the role that ageing persons fulfil as a community of wounded healers. In the second I shall consider disabled people from the perspective of wounds and healing. In the third section it will then be possible to sketch elements of an ethic that is attentive to the woundedness and healing that characterize the lives of persons who are elderly or who live with a disability.

Ageing persons: a community of wounded healers

From a theological viewpoint two notions are pivotal to any consideration of human ageing. The first is that we are embodied individuals. Throughout our lives we frequently ignore our bodiliness, when we are young and/or healthy. As the body increasingly becomes a locus of limits or pain it grabs our attention. The unity of body and spirit, or what came to be viewed in the post-Enlightenment era as the unity of body and mind, is a fragile one. At different times in our lives our bodies become something other – a machine to be kept in good running order (frequently the focus of the healthy ageing agenda), a commodity or a piece of private property (over which we exercise choice in areas such as sexuality and relationships, abortion or euthanasia), or a battleground (on which we fight disease or disability); when we are very old, it may become a prison that burdens our diminishing powers.

Accounts by disabled writers 'teach us that the serious diminution of any primary sense radically changes people's understanding of the physical world, of the interactions with other people, and of their conception of themselves' (May 1986, p.50). This is the wisdom of wounded healers. It has something to say to ageing persons as they encounter the disabling effects of chronic illness, mental frailty or simply the aches and pains of advancing age.

An understanding of ourselves as embodied persons is central to this chapter. It applies both to the fact that we age and to the disabilities associated with our later years. Post-Enlightenment Western culture is liberal in its world-view, assumptions, and expectations. Liberalism emphasizes the importance of reason, rationality, independence and the capacity for self-advocacy. Authentic human living presupposes a level of thinking and rationality necessary for the lives of free and independent equals who choose to associate. To be a person in this milieu is to be able to live one's life, develop one's potential and develop a purposeful life-course without reference to others. At centre stage in the liberal universe stands the independent, rational, autonomous individual (Swinton 2004). It has been well said by Stephen Post that 'clarity of mind and economic productivity determine the value of human life' (Post 2000). Any absence of these characteristics in the individual person places him or her outside the normal range and therefore disables them.

Hospitality encapsulates an *at-homeness* in the individual and an openness to the unexpected guest. This points to the second key notion, namely the role that friendship has in human living. The gift of self and the response of another in friendship far exceed the liberal focus on the autonomous individual. Friendship is possible no matter how able or disabled the participants are. A lifetime of friendships and their progressive loss in the later years are significant elements in the life journey of many elderly persons. Friendships enrich and enliven lives that are, at times, increasingly limited by diminished sight, hearing and mobility, and by burdens such as arthritis and the loss of mental acuity which accompanies the onset of dementia.

A network of friends gives depth and texture to lives experiencing loss and disappointment and gives to ageing persons the capacity to form community. As they contribute to community building they bring the strengths and weaknesses of character honed over decades. Whether enjoying good health or experiencing the limits that increase with the years, ageing individuals can contribute to social life by example that is virtuous. William F. May observes that

> [s]ome common human virtues – which men and women of all ages might do well to cultivate – simply take special form in the later years. When they do appear in the elderly, however, they can instruct and sometimes even inspire. Their example can encourage particularly the fainthearted among the young who believe that full human existence is possible only under the accidental circumstances of their own temporary flourishing. (May 1986, p.50)

May suggests that the virtue of courage should be seen to be the first in any list of virtues that might be attributed to ageing persons. I would go further and suggest that exercising the virtue of hospitality understood as at-homeness with self and openness to the other entails considerable courage and commitment at a time in a person's life when much changes and the reality of one's death is near.

Disabled people, wounds and healing

The Australian Disability Discrimination Act (1992), in line with similar legislation in other parts of the world, prohibits both direct and indirect discrimination against persons on the grounds of disability. It seeks to provide a mechanism for rectifying situations when discrimination does occur. The 1992 Act offers a broad notion of disability. It includes physical, intellectual, psychiatric, sensory, neurological and learning disabilities. It also includes physical disfigurement and the presence in the body of disease-causing organisms such as HIV. Current disabilities, together with those experienced in the past and any disabilities an individual may have in the future, fall under the scope of the legislation. Protection is also given to relatives, friends, carers and co-workers of people with disabilities.

Facts regarding disability in Australia

During the last twenty years the proportion of persons living with a disability has reached 17.1 per cent of the Australian population, a total of 3.3 million people. These people are usually restricted in carrying out one or more daily activities in areas such as care of self, mobility and communication. These restrictions are called 'core activity restrictions'. A number of factors contribute to this increase in the disabled population. First, people now are living longer lives and acquire disabilities as they age. Second, individuals who have had pre-existing disabilities are living longer. Third, social attitudes have changed enabling people to feel more comfortable about identifying themselves as having a disability (Australian Institute of Health and Welfare 2000a).

The notion 'disability' applies to a wide range of limitations. For some time *impairment* has been viewed as distinct from disability. The latter in turn is distinguished from *handicap* (Maddox 2001). Understandings of these three terms are much contested. As mentioned earlier the rate of disability increases as individuals age. While the proportion of males and females with disability is in general similar, disability rates vary across age groups. Among the disabled, elderly females aged 80 years and over have a much higher rate of disability than males of the same age (52% compared to 34%). This has obvious practical implications for the provision of aged care.

Biblical teaching and disability

Justice in the Bible is concerned with right relationships, with the 'restoration of a situation or environment which promotes equity and harmony in a community' (Freedman 1992). For the prophet Isaiah justice was a prerequisite for peace or *shalom* (Isaiah 65:17–25). The struggles Israel had in establishing its identity and place in the ancient Near East focused on the temple and practices of temple worship. It was only through the harsh experience of exile that Israel came to an awareness that justice and inclusive relationships are ultimately more important than temple worship (Isaiah 1:12–17). In both Old and New Testament periods what was designated as clean or unclean, and thus ritually pure or impure, functioned as a prism through which the individual or the community came to be seen. Leviticus 21:16–23 established the principle that bodily disability was to be considered an indication of cultic impurity. This mindset underpinned the reaction of the religious leaders to Jesus' cure of the man born blind in John 9.

The healing narratives in the gospels have an important role for they show how the established boundaries were crossed. Jesus touched the flesh of the leper (Mark 1:41) and laid hands on the woman doubled over (Luke 13:13). In the pagan territories the daughter of the Syro-Phoenician woman was cured (Mark 7:24–30), as were the demoniac (Mark 5:1–20) and the centurion's servant (Matthew 8:5–13). These healing miracles redefine the borders of God's rule. As Donald Senior well puts it, 'Jesus challenges the prescribed boundaries of God's people and demands access on behalf of those who have been excluded. The act of healing and transformation becomes an act of solidarity and inclusion' (Senior 1995, p.12).

The healing miracles in the ministry of Jesus alert us to an important distinction. As consumers of what modern medicine and health care have to offer, we hope for a cure when disease afflicts us. Cure is today understood primarily in a physical sense. The biblical notion of healing, on the other hand, goes well beyond achieving a physical cure. It gives priority to the spiritual transformation that occurs as the individual is cured. This explains why Jesus on a number of occasions directs the person who has been cured to go to the priests and have their healing verified. This ensured they could return to full life in the community. Not only is the cured person transformed by what has taken place but their cure also has an impact on the life and worship of the community.

Historical perspectives on disability

Theological reflection on the place of the poor and the weak in the human community provided a basis for Christian attitudes to disabled persons. From New Testament times they were seen to be passive recipients of a charity extended to those less blessed than the majority in the community. However, it is interesting in this context to note that the same standards were not applied to widows and orphans who very early became the first pastoral concern of the young Christian church. Many references exhort widows to live responsibly and contribute to the spiritual and material life of the community.

During the centuries that followed a range of responses may be observed in the West regarding the place of persons with disabilities. In the Middle Ages disabled people were viewed as a deviant group within society and thus judged to be second-class citizens (Eiesland 1994). By the seventeenth century, however, a marked change may be observed, for disabled persons by then were numbered among the 'deserving' poor who might have worked but for their impairments (Silvers 1996). More recently the increasingly dominant medical model of care has emphasized the idea of an impairment as a pathological condition (a genetic flaw, a chronic or acute disease, or an injury) that potentially compromises the capacity of an individual to carry out essential physiological, psychological or social tasks (Maddox 2001). Where a cure is no longer medically attainable, disability comes to be accepted as an involuntary and immutable state of affairs. For this way of thinking an *impairment* is viewed as an abnormal state in the individual. It follows, then, that *disability* came to refer to the compromised functioning that follows on an impairment. Use of the word *handicap* adds distinctly social and environmental dimensions to the experience of impairment and disability.

The medical approach to disability reinforced a common perception that to have a disability is a tragedy for the individual so afflicted (MacIntyre 1999). Some claim that this attitude is grounded in an irrational fear that healthy people have that they will themselves, at some time in the future, experience the burdens of disability. Furthermore, it is reinforced by the widespread perception that disability always involves dependence and abnormality. The reality is quite different. Being a disabled person is not necessarily a tragic state of affairs. Often the experience of disabled persons, their enjoyment of life, and even their identity and self-awareness as disabled is completely overlooked or discounted in the scheme of things (French and Swain 2002). Disability, after all, 'has social, experiential and biological components, present and recognized in different measures for different people' (Wendell 1989, p.108). It is vital to note that a physical condition, for example, may be viewed as disabling depending on time and place, social expectations, the current state of technology and its availability, the educational system, the built environment, attitudes towards physical appearance, and the pace of life (Wendell 1989).

Disability activists have strenuously rejected the medical model just sketched. They point to various barriers that contribute to institutionalized discrimination within society such as structures in the built environment and prevailing attitudes. It is certainly true that social factors play a significant role and add to the limits imposed on an individual by specific impairments. To enter further into debates presently under way in the area of disability studies would take us beyond the topics central to this chapter. It is sufficient to note by way of conclusion that all contributors to debates about disability give priority to the meaning that the experience disability has in the lives of persons living with a disability (French and Swain 2002).

Disabled persons challenge church communities today in two ways. Jean Vanier, when he speaks out of the rich experience of living in a L'Arche community, emphasizes the central place that human fulfilment has for the individual. Everyone desires that they flourish and have a sense of being fulfilled. He argues that it 'is realized in the way we use our capacities and our knowledge for other people's growth' (Vanier 2004, p.29). People who live with disabilities can teach us to be human. In doing this they lead the church to be an inclusive community. The second contribution that persons with disability make to the life of the church is to be found in the awareness that the church does not so much need to learn how to minister to disabled people but rather to be open to being ministered to and ultimately healed by them (Senior 1995). This will only occur when the hospitality that wounded healers can bring about is effective in the community of believers.

Ethics, ageing and disability

Hospitality and solidarity

The political contribution of disability activists has borne fruit in our Australian Disability Discrimination Act of 1992. In seeking to overcome discriminatory behaviour the hope is that as a civil society we will be more inclusive in the areas of everyday life and practice. At present 'Australian values' are being subjected to close scrutiny in public discourse. Should greater attention ever be given to ageing and disability in our society it would be possible to enrich the prevailing understanding of human interconnectedness and cohesion in ways not possible when the prevailing values of liberalism hold sway. The notion of solidarity 'highlights in a particular way the intrinsic social nature of the human person, the equality of all in dignity and rights and the common path of individuals and peoples towards an ever more committed unity' (Pontifical Council for Justice and Peace 2005, n.192). In our global village the interconnectedness of peoples is not only a social principle; it must also be expressed as a moral virtue.

Hospitality – a way beyond justice

Earlier it was noted that disabled persons were viewed as the passive recipients of charity offered to them by the able-bodied majority in society. Legislation that attempts to fight discrimination and prejudice fulfils a double role – it helps to shield individuals and groups from harm and at the same time seeks to promote their good. Two values make important contributions to this process. The first is justice, the second is participation. Right relationships are the core of the biblical understanding of justice. Giving each person their due raises the questions of whether (a) equal or equivalent treatment is to be offered, or (b) the route of preferential treatment implemented as affirmative action should be pursued (Kopelman 1996). When disabled persons are involved equality is foundational. Should significant inequalities exist then a case could well be made for preferential treatment. These issues are frequently played out when our duty as a civil society to provide appropriate care for ageing persons and persons with disabilities comes into conflict with the limits necessarily associated with resource allocation.

A focus on justice and resource allocation, while important, brings with it the danger of blinding us to other ethical principles equally important for our social lives. In the case of ageing and disability the principle of participation needs to be given emphasis. Participation

> is expressed essentially in a series of activities by means of which the citizen, either as an individual or in association with others, whether directly or through representation, contributes to the cultural, economic, political and social life of the civil community to which he (or she) belongs. (Pontifical Council for Justice and Peace 2005, n.189)

The right to participate in all aspects of the life of a society is grounded in the dignity of the human person and in that person's radically social nature. Being able to participate is thus an expression of the fundamental value that each human being is. It is essential to their identity and cannot be diminished by criteria based solely on capacity or functionality. Participation creates the possibility for a hospitality that crosses any boundaries that exist in a society.

Hospitality, dependence, and the common good

A fear of being dependent on others threatens all those who aspire to live their lives in terms of the liberal standard of being rational, autonomous individuals. To this way of thinking ageing and disability attack the integrity of the person. This prevailing fear may only be overcome when we can come to appreciate that, as human beings, we are all at some point on a continuum of dependence throughout all the stages of our human existence. In fact to realize our radical dependence makes it possible for us to recognize our interdependence as human beings and children of God. In this way of thinking 'dependence, vulnerability, and weakness are recognized not as deficits, but as a valued fundamental theological truth' (Swinton 2004). For Christians living under the sign of the cross it is possible to see that true independence is only possible in the experience of dependence. During much of our busy adult lives we tend to forget or even ignore this paradox of human existence.

A renewed appreciation of our dependence and interdependence is possible when we exercise the virtue of hospitality. It moves us beyond the individualism of the liberal worldview to a conviction that we have something to contribute to the common good. The 'principle of the common good, to which every aspect of social life must be related if it is to attain its fullest meaning, stems from the dignity, unity and equality of all people' (Pontifical Council for Justice and Peace 2005, n.164). The common good is understood as 'the sum total of social conditions which allow people, either as groups or as individuals, to reach their fulfilment more fully and more easily' (Flannery 1977, *Gaudium et spes*, n.26).

A society committed to the common good has the good of all people and the good of the whole person as its primary goal (Pontifical Council for Justice and Peace 2005, n.165). Human fulfilment and human flourishing are possible only when persons exist 'with' and 'for' others. This is most clearly exemplified in the hospitality that is shown to the aged and disabled in our society.

Conclusion

In this chapter I have chosen to explore the topic of ageing, disability, and ethics through the prism of hospitality. In doing so I have attempted to place the analysis of ageing, disability, and ethics in a larger context.

In human ageing we see the possibilities for the exercise of hospitality by wounded healers and the ways in which virtuous elderly persons have an exemplary and transformative role in society. In exploring the significance of disability, it has been possible to see the role of persons living with disability as alerting society at large to our human brokenness, dependence and interdependence.

As a theological ethicist I have utilized three basic principles of Catholic social-justice teaching in examining the issue at hand. In solidarity we are not only called to acknowledge the fact that we are interdependent with all others but also challenged to appreciate that it is a moral imperative for everyday life. In this sense it is truly the moral virtue for a globalized world. When focusing on the imperative for all citizens to participate in every aspect of our common social life the starting point is our nature as social beings. Societies where individuals or particular groups are hindered in their effort to participate in social life are fundamentally flawed. In acknowledging the central role played by the common good it has been possible to broaden our understanding of ageing and disability beyond the narrow confines imposed by the contemporary ethos of our liberal democratic societies. A hospitality that welcomes all as friends has the potential to overcome any barriers that marginalize elderly persons or individuals living with disability.

CHAPTER 4

New and Old Challenges of Ageing: Disabilities, Spirituality and Pastoral Responses

Elizabeth MacKinlay

Introduction

In recent years we have become much more aware of the issues surrounding mental health in later life. Dementia, in particular, and depression have gained higher focus and interest. Other chapters in this book range broadly across these topics. The biomedical model of disease has been criticized and an approach to care based on personhood and the value of the person, no matter what disabilities they encounter in their daily lives, has been strongly promoted.

A couple of years ago I was presenting a paper in which I outlined the model of spiritual tasks and process of ageing that I had developed in my doctoral studies (MacKinlay 1998, 2001a). Afterwards, over tea, a member of the audience approached me and said 'You know, this model is not just about ageing, but it fits those living with disabilities too.' She went on to speak of her child who had Down syndrome. I responded that my data were based on older adults, but that the model probably did fit those with disability too, whatever their age.

Since then I have had further similar conversations with others also connected with people who have disabilities, and I have reflected further on my data and the experience of living with Down's and other intellectual disabilities. The conference on which this book is based was one outcome of those conversations and reflections.

Back in the 1970s I became aware of the numbers of children with Down syndrome who were living at home and attending the local primary school; my daughter was in the same year at school as these children. This was in a rural community, where a group of these children were being mainstreamed in education. I believe this close contact with those children was valuable experience for the other children who learnt and played beside them.

Families then strived to keep their children with intellectual disabilities at home. It was seen as the 'right thing to do'. Now, several decades on, we see these children, now adult children, living longer than was generally the case in previous generations. However, now further challenges arise, as these ageing adult children with intellectual disabilities and their own ageing parents struggle with the patterns of a lifetime, seeking to adjust to ageing together. Ageing people with lifelong disabilities like Down syndrome and cerebral palsy have complex health needs, often involving physical as well as psychological and spiritual aspects. How we relate to these people makes a critical difference to their overall well-being. Christine Bigby (2004) notes that these people are often further disadvantaged in society as they have been unable to earn or at least earn sufficient during their earlier lives to be able to save for their retirement.

While I was writing this I received a letter from a widow underlining the importance of recognizing the need for care of older people with disabilities. Fay Brassington had seen the advertisement for the Centre for Ageing and Pastoral Studies (CAPS) conference on the opposite page to her husband's obituary in the diocesan newspaper, the *Anglican News*. Len Brassington had been a priest. I have Fay's permission to include part of her letter and I think it is very relevant to our topic.

My husband who spent his working life at the core of the caring professions developed a rare frontal lobe dementia some years ago and ended his days mute and immobile and in need of total care. Despite this I believe he performed his most enduring ministry during this time. Through his condition our children and grandchildren learnt acceptance and compassion, I became more patient and tolerant and all who visited our home – nurses, therapists, carers and friends were uplifted. As one council carer wrote after his death

> As a carer it was a privilege to take care of Len, as a friend it was a blessing to have known such a gentle, kind and loving soul. He may never have uttered a single word to me but he taught me a really valuable life's lesson. He taught me how to just 'be' with another human being.

Of course this says as much about the carer as the cared for but it illustrates that age and disability need not be any less satisfying and worthwhile than any other stage of life.

Throughout my husband's latter years we experienced daily 'resurrections' and minor miracles and although he couldn't say so I believe his life was happy. However, surprisingly, the one thing lacking during these years was any spiritual contact from the local or diocesan clergy.

This is not meant to be a criticism as changes in clergy and my husband's ongoing condition over many years made continuity of care quite difficult. And as we had clergy and lay friends, our own inner resources and access to radio and TV religious programs I have no cause to complain. However others may not be as fortunate. Isolation and loneliness as you know is a major problem for the disabled aged and their carers and to be cut off from the local faith community can leave a big void in one's spiritual life.

To provide a ministry to the disabled aged may be difficult when there appears to be little or no response. But because of something that happened in our situation I know that such ministry is well worth working towards.

Eighteen months before his death my husband developed cancer and it was then that regular visitation and communion was re-instated. Communion days saw my husband more alert. He fought to stay awake, following the service with his eyes and even on occasion took the bread in his hand (a hand that hadn't moved for several years). Any improvement in my husband's condition lifted my spirits also so the ministry was doubly valuable.

Without being judgemental (only personal experience has en-lightened me) the fact that the church showed love and compassion when cancer occurred suggests there is an understanding of illness that doesn't necessarily extend to disability and ageing.

Fay ended the letter by writing that she is excited at knowing of conferences such as this one and hopes for positive outcomes. May we not disappoint her!

In this chapter I will reflect on the challenges of living with disabilities and ask some questions, few of which draw immediate answers. These questions are related to issues of personhood, of relationship and acceptance of people living with disabilities. I will write of intellectual disabilities that people have lived with all their lives, and of acquired disabilities of ageing that present challenges for older people. I will not be focusing on the disabilities themselves, but rather on the effects of the disabilities for spirituality in ageing. Further I want to ask, can the model that I designed for spiritual tasks of ageing be used to help understand the issues of ageing and disabilities, whatever the origin of disability?

Living with lifelong disabilities and ageing: families and ageing with Down syndrome

What are these long-term relationships of people with Down syndrome and their families based on? First, they are based on mutual acceptance and love, but also interlaced with the struggles for understanding of each other. Communication is just one area where particular problems may emerge, complicating adequate understandings of both the parents and the adult children who have Down syndrome.

Then there are the struggles for acceptance of the family and the person with the disability by the wider community. Is the person with Down's treated as a person, with feelings, needs and a spirituality of their own? Are these people afforded a sense of dignity and appropriate care and support by others? Do the communities of faith realize the importance of faith to those who have intellectual disabilities? Do our communities of faith affirm the worth and dignity of these people? Continuing community education is required to prevent stereotyping, to prevent repeatedly underestimating what the person is capable of, and denying them an identity.

As part of my research into ageing and disability, I met with the brother and sister-in-law of Michael who had Down syndrome and had lived until age 66. The interview was audio-taped and transcribed. In the interview they described the latter years of their brother's life. Michael's brother said: 'So we are looking at someone who had a 60-year lifespan, though he died at the age of 66. At the end of his life he was blind and he was deaf and he was demented.' Michael's sister-in-law didn't agree that Michael was demented, but thought that he was terrified and this then resulted in a type of behaviour that could best be described as 'demented'. By way of explanation she said: 'The sort of patterns of light that hit his now blind eyes quite suddenly, I think that what he described was not madness, but actually what it felt like, to be where he was at that time.'

When we have not experienced something ourselves, and it is different from anything we can imagine, we may seek to explain whatever it is by labelling it, or perhaps by rejecting the authenticity of the experience. There is a natural human tendency to separate ourselves from what we cannot understand. Yet something more is asked of us, and that is to be with people who are vulnerable and who live with disabilities. By being with them, we can be part of life's journey towards wholeness, both for the person with disability and also for our own growth towards wholeness.

People who have Down syndrome and are older now are part of the cohort who lived through times where the condition was not well understood, when often the person with Down's was kept in an institution and not expected to live long. They were certainly not regarded as being capable of benefiting from education. Their often multiple health problems not infrequently resulted in a short life. Now, however, this has changed markedly and many more people with Down's are living longer. What happens when they are in need of care and the parents who have cared for them all their lives are growing older and less capable of providing adequate care? Eileen Glass addresses many of these issues in Chapter 5.

Acquired disabilities of ageing

Depression too is commonly found among older people. Fleming (2001a), in a national study, found that approximately 50 per cent of people admitted to residential aged care in Australia were depressed. Depression is still too often seen as a normal part of growing old. Issues of isolation and loneliness certainly operate in increasing the prevalence of depression in these people.

With regard to people who live with dementia, whatever its cause, too often the focus is on eliminating the disease and maybe the person as they become labelled as the disease. Christine (Boden 1998; Bryden 2005) (see Chapter 11, pp.135–144) was first diagnosed as having early onset Alzheimer's in the mid 1990s. Later this diagnosis was revised to fronto-temporal dementia. Christine has been quite remarkable in her fight for justice and recognition of the person with dementia. She is an international speaker, although she is accepting fewer speaking invitations now. One person working in the area of policy in ageing discounted Christine's witness by saying 'well she hasn't got Alzheimer's she's got fronto-temporal dementia, therefore she can't speak for people with Alzheimer's'. I would dismiss that assertion as irrelevant, since dementia, whatever its label, has effects that are hard to live with and tend to isolate those who live with that diagnosis.

The diagnosis of dementia or the fact of living with an intellectual disability can not only be hard for the person whose life it is, but may also have an adverse effect on others – family, friends, and community. A medical practitioner recently diagnosed with Alzheimer's told me that he had decided to tell his colleagues of his diagnosis, and as a result he now felt rejected by them.

I would say that what is operating in these situations is fear. Fear is the opposite of love. Fear can be paralysing and shut people out, isolating them. We know this in other spheres in our current society, where people who are deemed to be different from us are excluded. This is a fear that drives terrorism. It is fear that keeps people who are different from the accepted norm, separated from others.

Perfect love, the love of God, casts out fear. This begs the question for us, who are less than God, how do we love what may seem to be unlovable? How do we move from fear to love?

What are the factors that operate, at least to some extent, in these situations of people with disabilities: intellectual, or dementia, or even depression?

- *Fear and misunderstanding*
  Fear will lead to misunderstanding as people withdraw or separate from contact with the thing or person feared. Fear grows and the object feared becomes further separated and therefore less known. Knowledge and experience can help lessen fear. Sometimes we are afraid to venture into new and unknown situations. When Christine asked me to walk a journey into dementia with her as her spiritual adviser, I was fearful. My biomedical model informed through years of nursing wanted to say 'no' to her request. I wanted to run, anywhere but into being so close to someone who had dementia. But I prayed and knew then that I was to journey with her. Apart from any support that I might have given to Christine, this has been an enriching experience for me and it has informed much of what I have done since, in regard to my practice as a clergy person and as a nurse. Further, it has formed the direction of research that I have engaged in and with.

- *Seeking answers to everything*
  Normal human curiosity leads people to seek answers to everything, to be able to label everything. A worldview that sees the biomedical model as the only option may prevent seeing other ways and other answers, or even the possibility to live without answers. In a way, the biomedical model, although valuable in many ways, blinds us to using other lenses to see reality, and to be able to live with mystery and the unknown.

- *Seeking cure rather than wholeness and healing*
  The twentieth-century view was to cure all diseases. Largely, we are still operating from within that mode. The more important thing is to

journey with people and to grow towards wholeness and healing, rather than cure. It is told that St Francis overcame his fear of leprosy by embracing a leper. Is this a lesson from long ago that we can adopt in our care? When we meet the fearful situation or the person feared, can we reach out to the person instead of turning away? In moving toward the person or thing feared, the fear seems to fall away.

The model of spiritual tasks and process of ageing

How can we apply a model of spiritual tasks of ageing to working with those who are growing older and live with disabilities? Out of this model (MacKinlay 2001a) I want to draw on all six components. I would normally put the finding of ultimate meaning as the first component of the model, before relationship, but it is apparent from our studies that, for people with dementia, relationship is almost synonymous with meaning. Further, the term connectedness seems to more adequately describe relationship for people with dementia. The second component of the model is the search for and finding of ultimate meaning. The third component of the model is the move from provisional life meanings, to finding final meanings. Vulnerability which increases with disability and ageing presents a fourth task of the model that is identified as the struggle towards transcendence.

Often, for people living with disabilities, it is the response to meaning that entails the use of symbols, ritual, and liturgy, that helps to bring the whole spiritual and religious experience into a meaningful event for them. The fifth component is the need for symbol and ritual. Out of these components springs the sixth component, hope.

Connectedness

In all our in-depth interviews with people with dementia, the need for connectedness was evident. Even for those with low Mini Mental State Examination (MMSE) scores and with little speech, there was still a need for connection with others. A problem that emerges for some is the difficulty of establishing that connectedness. Speech may be limited; family may have trouble in understanding the person and carers may be too busy to allow time to hear what the person is endeavouring to communicate.

Perhaps even then fear gets in the way of really reaching out to these people. It may be easier to say, 'she doesn't know who I am' and so find a reason we don't have to try. So many people, when they know my mother is in a nursing home and has dementia, ask 'Does she recognize you?' I think that is the wrong question. Here I turn to the work of Tom Kitwood (1997) as he defined personhood, and put the onus on carers and family to reach out to the person with dementia, to bestow dignity and personhood on them, rather than expecting the person with dementia to initiate the conversation, based on whether we think they 'know who we are'.

Some so-called 'difficult behaviours' can be strategies that endeavour to gain needed attention of loved ones or staff. Too often we use the term 'attention-seeking' as if it was a bad word. People who have problems in communicating need to get attention somehow! If we are too busy or not open to their needs, then the need may escalate in urgency. Sometimes we are just too tired, too stressed to even notice until the 'behaviour' has become a crisis.

The search for life meaning

Life without meaning results in despair, hopelessness and sometimes the desire for the final solution of ending it all – for suicide. Humans are meaning-makers; part of the spiritual dimension is the searching for meaning, the desire to connect with ultimate meaning (Frankl 1984; Kimble 1990, 2003; MacKinlay 2001a). The search for ultimate meaning is influenced by the person's ability to form deep and significant relationships. It is influenced, more often in later life, by the ability to transcend the disabilities and losses encountered in the life journey. The search is influenced by the ability of the person to find symbols and ritual that connect them with their source of ultimate meaning, for example, through worship. Music, art, and environment are also important triggers in facilitating meaning and a sense of awe. People who have disabilities may find it difficult to find meaning when loved ones have died, or when they are moved to live in residential care. Communication difficulties may compound their struggle to find meaning. Yet, at some level, the search for meaning is still there.

The search for final life meanings

I want to distinguish between the search for meaning that is present throughout human life and the search for final meanings that occurs in the face of impending mortality.

Through all of our lives we seek to know the meaning of events and circumstances. This will be unconscious at times, and at other times that search will become very real and central in one's life. This is a feature of being in a suicidal situation, experiencing suicidal ideation; the person can no longer find that sense of meaning and purpose in their lives.

During most of our lives, we assign provisional meaning to situations (Frankl 1984) while, when faced with our own impending mortality, we may perhaps, for the first time seek the real and final meaning of our lives. That is, in the best of circumstances. For some, to even begin to seek final meaning may be perceived as too painful.

COMING TO FINAL MEANINGS: IDENTITY THROUGH STORY

Narrative provides us with the sense of our identity. This is basic to being human. For Christians, our story is interlaced with God's story and the story of our community of faith.

Kenyon (Kenyon, Clark and de Vries 2001) has written that we are story. As we age that story becomes more important and the questions 'Who am I?' and 'What has my life been worth?' grow in importance.

As we have worked with people who have dementia we have heard them say 'I don't have a story – I am just an ordinary person' (Trevitt and MacKinlay 2006). We all have a story that revolves around and informs our identity. If that story can be told, then that has power for healing, for growing towards wholeness and integrity. The people with dementia did tell their stories; they did connect with their lives and meaning. For Christians, this story is made whole through realizing not just our own story, but the connections of the story with our families, our communities of faith and our story with God. This connection is missing in the wider society, where people do not want to see the whole, but only wish to engage in a postmodern perspective of relativism.

Transcendence and unpredictability

One of the challenges of the journey into later life for many people is unexpected and previously unknown disabilities and illnesses. While in earlier life a person can be pretty sure that they can plan ahead and make commitments, in later life disabilities can flare suddenly, and this gives rise to a sense of loss of control over one's life.

People who have been highly independent during most of their adult lives may suddenly find themselves at a new place, and a place they may not like. Even Bill Clinton, arriving at age 60 – not really old at all – admitted to not liking being that age.

Unpredictability becomes part of life; it is the fear of going out of control that many older people living independently expressed in earlier studies (MacKinlay 2001b). This gives rise to the sense of vulnerability, as distinct from self-sufficiency. Each meeting with a health crisis brings one back to that precise moment of the day; it is not possible to plan ahead, or sometimes it is not possible to know how one is going to get through this one day.

But each time, when this crisis has passed, the person finds themselves in a different place. For some people, wisdom is growing, and a letting-go may be taking place. On the other hand, the person may come out of the crisis frightened and withdraw into themselves. It is the members of this latter group who may feel relief when they are admitted to an aged care facility, where they can know help is available. How do we support these older people in their anxieties and fears experienced through health crises, and through just losing their abilities to do what they once were able to do?

In a society that affirms people for 'doing', for outcomes, for achievements, there is little affirmation for those who 'cannot do'. Those who can no longer contribute in tangible ways to society are cast off and devalued. Communities of faith that offer a different way of living can do much to support these people. Often in our busy churches, as well as the wider society, those who can no longer 'do' or be involved in activities are forgotten and become the 'shut-ins' perhaps living alone with few social contacts. Often these older people have few or no family to support them. I have spoken with many of these people in recent years, people who acutely feel the loneliness and isolation and who feel cut off from their church communities and pastoral care. Sometimes the failure to reach out to those who are more frail and/or housebound is because of the busyness of those who are not disabled. Even those who provide pastoral care seem stretched and unable to take on more care. There seems to be no time to remember those who are disabled. Another case that illustrates the potential for being isolated at home was the man I have written about earlier in this chapter, who had dementia, and then was diagnosed with cancer.

Ritual and symbol

Symbols help all of us to connect to meaning, and to experience a sense of awe, if the symbols are right. We are meaning-makers; and often people who live with disabilities and who have no speech find symbols even more important; as shown in Len Brassington's action as he moved his hand to hold the bread during communion. The symbols and the rituals help make the connections. Emotion, feelings and spirituality are carried by the rituals and the use of symbols in these. Music, art and dance are important bearers of meaning, especially for those who struggle to find the right words to express what they want to say.

Hope

Hope is not a task of ageing so much as a coming to 'being' that arises, often out of the other tasks of ageing. We can't 'do' hope. However, we may become hopeful through life experiences or even through a letting-go of a difficult situation and relying on a source of strength outside of ourselves. Hope may be present in the seemingly most hopeless of circumstances (Frankl 1984).

Hope is possible:

- when the person finds meaning and purpose in their being
- through the examining of a life and its story
- when a person transcends a seemingly insurmountable situation
- when a person believes in a god of love.

Conclusion

Identifying and addressing both new and old challenges of ageing and disabilities is actually quite simple. It is not rocket science. We know how to do this.

But further than that, to actually do it becomes complex. We meet with all sorts of challenges.

- It costs too much, both for churches and the wider society.
- We have to put our resources into youth ministry, the 'hope of the future', and there is not enough to go round. This leaves little hope for youth as they will see only too clearly that when they grow older, they too will be cast off.
- It is not seen as attractive to work with disabled and older people. There is stigma attached to age and even more so to disabled old people.
- We are still fearful of age and disabilities.
- We take on the values of the secular society that wants cure and quick fixes.
- That does not work with older and disabled people.
- We don't have the will to do it.

Imagine a new world, a world where people are valued because they are made in God's image. This would mean a world:

- that affirms people with disabilities and mental illness
- where age is valued as much as youth
- where we encourage strong connections between young people and older people, disabled or not
- that affirms being, not just doing.

This would be heaven.

Can we not have heaven on earth? Surely this is the model that Jesus left for us. But then, the Beatitudes have always been an awful challenge for human beings.

CHAPTER 5

The Particular Needs of Older People with Intellectual Disabilities and Their Carers: A Perspective from the Experience of L'Arche

Eileen Glass

Introduction

In exploring the needs of older people with intellectual disabilities and the contribution they can make to the conversation about ageing, disability and spirituality, I am writing from the perspective of having shared my life with people with intellectual disabilities for over thirty years. The context of my life sharing has been through my membership of L'Arche Winnipeg in Canada and L'Arche Genesaret in Canberra as well as from my work with communities in India, Japan, the Philippines and New Zealand.

I begin with a brief introduction to L'Arche and to the reality of living with an intellectual disability. I then outline the spirituality of L'Arche which underpins the principles and values on which L'Arche communities have based the development of support for people as they age and die. Throughout, I draw on examples from communities in different countries, using reflections of long-term assistants as they have accompanied ageing members in their need for increased support, their need to move to other settings, and in some instances through their process of dying.

Introducing L'Arche

The first community of L'Arche was founded in France in 1964. Our founder, Jean Vanier, had met people with intellectual disabilities in large institutions and realized that they were excluded from society because they were weak, and their need for support posed a question and a challenge to societies where strength and independence are dominant values. He discovered that people who are limited in their intellectual capacity exhibit a correspondingly developed capacity for relationship. He noticed that when he visited the institution, people asked relational questions: 'What's your name? Will you be my friend? Will you come and visit me again?' In comparison, the students to whom he was teaching philosophy at university were not as interested in his person as in his capacity: his capacity to enable them to pass their exams! Jean realized that what is most vulnerable in our humanity, our need and cry for authentic relationship, is pushed under in our striving for success, recognition and power.

We feel vulnerable when we are in touch with the cry in our own hearts, with the yearning to live out the fullness of who we are, free from the constraints of social and cultural expectations. In welcoming Raphael Simi and Philippe Seux to share his modest home in the village of Trosly Breuil, Jean hoped that in sharing life together they would experience a level of acceptance which would in turn enable them to become more accepting of their own disabilities. Jean was still to discover the part these men would play in his own healing and transformation. Jean's vision and the values it represents are given voice in the Charter of L'Arche:

> Whatever their gifts or limitations, people are all bound together in a common humanity. Everyone is of unique and sacred value, and everyone has the same dignity and the same rights. The fundamental rights of each person include the rights to life, to care, to a home, to education and to work. Also, since the deepest need of a human being is to love and to be loved, each person has a right to friendship, to communion and to a spiritual life. (Federation of L'Arche 1993, 11 Fundamental Principles 1)

The focus of L'Arche communities is to build relationships of friendship and mutuality through the creation of family-sized homes where people with disabilities and their assistants live together, sharing the tasks of home-making, and in some countries through participation in work projects. The training and competence assistants bring to the task of offering support to people with disabilities is always at the service of developing friendship. Since 1964 L'Arche has grown into a worldwide federation of 130 such communities in 33 countries and each new foundation is made through links with an existing community so that significant friendships are integral to the growth of L'Arche.

Living with an intellectual disability

Intellectual disability, by its nature, puts people outside the ambit of the dominant values of our culture; values of competence, efficiency, productivity, physical beauty; all that stems from the power of the intelligence and the myth of the perfect genetic makeup. People who do not function in terms of these values pose powerful questions about what it means to be human. Of what does our fundamental humanity consist? What is at the basis of our judgments about one another, our prejudices which drive us to deny fullness of humanity to each other? If we are truthful, we know that each one of us lives with one or more disabling conditions; however, we are taught from an early age to compensate for our inadequacies, to mask and deny them. We fall victim to a value system which ranks people as being of more or less importance depending on their capacity, rather than on their inherent dignity as human persons. We become terrified of any incapacity or limitation in our own lives and we live with the fear of being found out.

We know that from the moment of our birth we begin the journey towards ageing and death. We are grateful if we are accorded a long and fruitful journey, though we grieve the passage itself as it brings increasing diminishment and often more than its share of pain. We might ask how much of the pain springs from the fact that we can no longer deny the reality of our disabilities. They are writ large for all to see and we are humbled as we are revealed for who we are. People who have lived with disabilities throughout their lives are often more accepting of the ageing process and adapt to it more gracefully than typical people who are making the adjustment to life with a disability acquired in later life.

One of the notable characteristics of many people with intellectual disability is their ease in entering into relationship with others. The Charter of L'Arche says:

> People with an intellectual disability often possess qualities of welcome, wonderment, spontaneity and directness. They are able to touch hearts and to call others to unity through their simplicity and vulnerability. In this way they are a living reminder to the wider world of the essential values of the heart without which knowledge, power and action lose their meaning and purpose. (Federation of L'Arche 1993, 11 Fundamental Principles 3)

In many ways people with an intellectual disability represent the human heart unmasked and they can startle us with their directness, their transparency and their deep compassion. The capacity to live from the heart assumes a particular importance in our later years as our time of productivity is over and our human task is to live more deeply in relationship with those around us. In this, people with an intellectual disability can help show us the way.

The spirituality of L'Arche

Jean Vanier's response to the cry of people in the institution was to create a community where each member, whatever their limitations or their gifts, would have a valued place. His reading of the Gospel convinced him that the message of Jesus calls his followers to become friends with those on the margins of the dominant culture. Choosing to be a friend with a person who has been rejected or marginalized offers both a challenge and a profound possibility for mutual healing and growth. Friendship implies presence one to the other, readiness to spend time together. It is less about 'doing for' and more about 'being with'. It calls for an authenticity which is not afraid to reveal vulnerability and to grow in mutuality. Until I am able to truly receive from the other, to be challenged and enriched by the person who has a visible disability, I have not yet begun to build true friendship.

L'Arche has often been described as a Roman Catholic community. This description, while recognizing the spiritual milieu of the original foundation, fails to take account of the development of communities in different cultural and religious settings around the world. From the beginning L'Arche was clearly a spiritual as well as a therapeutic community:

> L'Arche communities are communities of faith, rooted in prayer and trust in God. They seek to be guided by God and by their weakest members, through whom God's presence is revealed. Each community member is encouraged to discover and deepen his or her spiritual life and live it according to his or her particular faith and tradition. Those who have no religious affiliation are also welcomed and respected in their freedom of conscience. (Federation of L'Arche 1993, 111 The Communities: Communities of Faith 1.1)

Wherever L'Arche communities have begun, it has always been with the focus of welcoming people who need a home, a place of friendship and support. The communities bring together people of different backgrounds and religious traditions and this diversity implies the task of building unity in the midst of difference. 'Communities recognize that they have an ecumenical vocation and a mission to work for unity' (Federation of L'Arche 1993, 111 The Communities: Communities of Faith 1.3). To build community in such circumstances requires a spirituality which speaks to the diversity of human experience and the reality of human limitation, and which gives meaning to life lived outside the affirmation of dominant cultural values.

Whatever the cultural or religious context of L'Arche communities, their spirituality is based in the Beatitudes of Jesus. The Beatitudes articulate a vision of God for humankind; they challenge us to find meaning in those aspects of human experience which the dominant culture devalues or seeks to deny. 'Blessed are the poor in spirit, …the gentle, …those who mourn, …who are persecuted, …who hunger and thirst for what is right' (Matthew 5:1–12). In valuing these dimensions of human experience we are led beyond the notion of a God who expects that our lives be perfect: perfectly whole, perfectly happy, or perfectly peaceful. We are given a language and a spirituality that speaks to the reality of lives which are limited, impoverished, marked by imperfection, grief, marginalization, and suffering. We are invited to discover the face of God present in such life experiences, and to dare to hope that they may offer a passage to growth, to transformation, to the wholeness that lies in accepting the diversity of human experience.

This hope is radically illustrated in a letter written by Kathy Baroody in July 2006. Kathy is a member of L'Arche living on the West Bank. The community of L'Arche in Bethany had to be closed at the time of the first Gulf War and Kathy has lived there for many years, to be a presence of L'Arche to community members who had to return to the institution and who might otherwise be alone, without hope. Kathy wrote:

> Our region is being shattered by the world's most powerful weapon: fear. Fear blinds and maims. It tortures and kills. It is the source of lies and destruction. It builds walls and prisons. It traumatizes children and sweeps adults into the pit of despair. And here I sit, in the relative, eerie calm of Bethlehem, struggling to make sense of what is going on around us. The horrors of Gaza are gathering relentless momentum. The systematic destruction of Lebanon has just begun. The Wall around Bethlehem is almost complete. And yet Ghadir, a young woman with severe physical and intellectual disabilities who lives in an institution in Bethany, still greets me with a belly laugh and sparkling eyes when I walk in the door. As she gracefully moves her hands up and down, I recognize her invitation to dance. And so we dance. Ghadir has lived her whole life knowing her limitations. She has encountered frustration and pain. She knows what it means to be gripped by fear. She knows what it feels like to be the source of fear for people who look at her and see someone less than human. Ghadir has somehow accepted the paralysis of her body. But she refuses to succumb to the paralysis of her heart. With the joy she wants to share and the thirst she has for friendship, she has discovered the weapons that

> destroy fear. She didn't spend years and years and billions of dollars on research. She simply realized that each moment is a gift, an invitation to enter into relationship with others. Ghadir has created a little world of peace. A little world where each person is welcomed. A little world of healing. A little world where gratitude is possible. Ghadir has invited me into this little world where hope becomes possible again. And because of Ghadir, I am able to invite others into this world of hope. (Baroody 2006)

Growing old together

When L'Arche began, the focus was on giving people a home for life, that is, a home where they would experience themselves as welcome, valued, and supported to grow according to their capacities and desires. It also meant that their home would be lifelong if that was what they wanted and if L'Arche was able to offer appropriate support for their changing needs. At that stage there was no clear understanding of what it might mean to accompany people to the end of life. We have had to learn about that as we went along and our learning has given rise to questions and insights we could not have anticipated thirty years ago. As assistants we have also had to engage with our own experience of ageing, of living with chronic illness or disability alongside our friends who have long borne the label of disability. As we go on together we discover new depths in the possibility for personal transformation which lie in the experience of growing older together.

Seniors programmes

In the mid 1980s, around twenty years after the beginning of L'Arche, some communities began to establish Seniors programmes for people who were no longer able to participate in work or other day programmes outside the L'Arche community. One of the first, the Seniors Club, was established in the Daybreak community in Toronto, Canada. I want to look at the principles underlying this programme and their practical application for people in L'Arche who are ageing (Zimmerman 1991).

Fecundity / fruitfulness

As people grow older they need to be cared for and affirmed in their place in the community; they also need to be supported to stay in touch with their inner selves, to discover that their lives remain a source of life for others and that they have the capacity to offer their lives for others and to God.

Activities in the Seniors Club which speak to this need include: helping out with community correspondence, as elders who hold much of the communal memory; hosting morning teas for people such as newcomers and visitors to the community; and visiting community members who are hospitalized. In this the Seniors offer a valuable service to building the life of their community.

Belonging

One of the sufferings of old age is the gradual shrinking of our friendship circle: our world narrows, our health becomes fragile, energy diminishes. Long-time friends age and some die. Everyone who joins the Seniors Club needs to have a sense of belonging, a place to relax with friends and enjoy conversation, to pursue interests and hobbies and to encourage and support one another in these endeavours. As a sense of belonging is enhanced, then self-esteem generally improves. With greater self-esteem people tend to be more motivated, more active and generally more satisfied.

Motivation and empowerment

People are encouraged to talk about how they would like to spend their retirement and are supported in following their choices. When invited to take personal responsibility and to make choices within realistic parameters, feelings of being valued and in control are enhanced. Some people look to the Seniors Club to enable them to engage in social activities, to pursue interests and for companionship. Others ask for support from the programme to do their shopping, keep appointments or prepare for visits to family and friends.

Rhythm of life

Life rhythms change with age; health needs have to be respected as changes occur in strength, stamina and endurance. Alternation of rest and activity, sedentary tasks and those requiring more physical exertion make for a more relaxed and comfortable day. Programme planning needs to be flexible and provision of a comfortable space where one can relax is important. People are encouraged to decide which activities best correspond with their energy levels at different times of the day.

Life issues/the life story

As people begin retirement and face the reality of growing older, there are often significant life issues which require attention. Many of these issues involve grief and loss: the death of parents and siblings, loss of mobility or sensory function, the need for major medical procedures. As such issues surface for individuals, time is given to address questions and concerns. At this point in the life of the person, it is important to be aware of the bigger picture of their life journey and so the Life Story Project developed.

This project is usually undertaken with a long-term friend who knows the person well. Over a period of many months there is a process of contacting family, friends and others who have been significant in the life of the person and inviting them to record their memories of the person. Photographs are collected and some people include their favourite songs, places they have travelled, important world events they can remember. The story records significant life transitions which have already been lived, as well as the story of the person's early years in the L'Arche community. All of this material is eventually collected into a book and there is often a ceremony of blessing the book; in effect blessing all of the life of the person.

The book may then be used in a variety of ways: it provides a resource for carers who may know little of the life story of the person; it can be used when speaking about L'Arche in different settings; it safeguards the story of the person as they become more vulnerable and less able to communicate in familiar ways.

The experience of the assistants in the Seniors programme

The Life Story Project is significant not only for the person concerned but also for the friend who accompanies the person in the project. We would all be familiar with the experience of discovering the life of a friend from a new perspective, of learning about experiences and accomplishments of which we were previously unaware. When we allow ourselves to be touched by the life of the other, we are always changed.

One of the people who helped establish the Seniors Club in Toronto expressed her experience in this way:

> We are invited to live with the eyes of faith, seeing the heart within the body which is gradually being stripped of its capacities. We are challenged to recognize that we are not our body, that the body's fecundity is surpassed by a deeper fecundity of the heart. We are invited to discover the meaning of relationship, a meaning that lies at the heart of God.

> Our people teach us that life is not what we do or what we have: it is not the strength of our body nor of our mind, nor the cleverness of our hands. It is not even our friends, nor our family and relationships. Rather its meaning is hidden in the heart of God, in the mystery of God who is life, from whom we come and to whom we go. (Zimmerman 1991)

One of the assistants currently working in the Seniors Club has been part of the programme for thirteen years. In writing about her friendship with Annie she says:

> My visits to Annie at the hospital the year before she died taught me the value of silence. Annie would welcome me to her hospital room like a long-lost friend. We would talk about all the people we knew in common. Then Annie would choose one of her books on the English royalty and I would start to knit. We would sit in silence for the next hour. It was such a gift to me, that quiet time in Annie's hospital room. (Kelly 2006)

L'Arche communities in the province of Ontario have developed a document entitled 'A Vision of Supporting Our Members with Intellectual Disability as they Age and Die' (L'Arche Ontario 2005). It names ten core values which underpin the support L'Arche seeks to offer to people who are growing older. I would like to explore some of these core values: relationships of mutuality, forgiveness and celebration, and emotional and spiritual support.

The therapy of L'Arche is essentially a therapy of relationship. We believe that by choosing to share life and build relationships of friendship, mutuality, celebration and forgiveness, we will experience healing and growth in wholeness. Our commitment to one another is that we will maintain these relationships for the whole life of the other person. This is not to say that there will not be significant change in the way the relationship is lived. People move on in their own lives but that does not imply the relationship itself is severed. When a person's needs change in such a way that it is no longer possible or appropriate for the person to remain in a L'Arche home, then care is taken to maintain the relationship within the context of a new setting.

In 2006 the community of L'Arche Sydney accompanied one of their members through her final illness to death. Pat Harper was a woman who was deeply loved in her own family and in L'Arche. Her question to each of us was always 'Do you love me?' and when we answered 'Yes, I do' she would say 'And I love you too'. This question, the same one that Jesus asked Peter after the resurrection as he called him to mission, was the central question of Pat's life. It expressed Pat's mission. She was like a beacon to all around her, calling us to the fundamental truth of our existence – to be loving people. Pat's spiritual accompanier through the time of her illness told me, 'When she said your name she took you into her heart and you knew that you were loved.' This person told me that at times she herself is afraid of the fact that she is growing older because there are still things she wants to do in her life. Her journey with Pat taught her something about surrender, about allowing life to unfold, not raging against what could not be changed.

When Pat was in the hospital and later in the hospice, people from her household would go every night to have their time of community prayer with her. This was an important way of holding Pat in the circle of her home life and of enabling the other members of the household to journey with her in a daily way. Maintaining the circle of friendship is important in enabling people to integrate the changing circumstances of their lives.

News of Pat's death reached a group of 46 members of L'Arche Australia who were on a pilgrimage to central Australia just as some of them assembled to watch the sunrise at Uluru. One pilgrim wrote:

> We were there at the Centre – at Uluru –
> On the day Pat asked God:
> 'Do you love me?'
> and
> God said, 'Come and see!' (Snudden 2006)

That afternoon our pilgrim band prayed for Pat at the Kata Tjutas and in the evening we drank a beer for her (she loved a beer) and danced with each other, knowing that Pat was dancing with God. Days later, when the pilgrims had returned home, community members, family and friends gathered to share memories and stories of Pat's life; this is the custom in L'Arche communities at a time of death. The night before her funeral she was brought home and people kept vigil with her. These rituals are important in enabling community members to mourn in appropriate ways, to begin to integrate the reality of the person's death, and to be assured that when their turn comes they too will be honoured and celebrated.

Maintaining a sense of home

Responding to the changing needs of the person may necessitate changes in the life of the home. This has consequences for everyone: the person concerned, and other members of the household, both people with disabilities and assistants. The introduction of physical aids will impact on space in bedrooms, bathrooms and living rooms; the need for therapists, palliative care personnel or other professionals to visit the house will affect the rhythm of daily life. Other people with disabilities living in the home may feel they are receiving less attention from the assistants. Assistants may need to acquire new skills and face questions about their own fragility and mortality as they journey with the person. It is not always easy to negotiate the complex needs which may arise on any given day.

Last year an older man in our community in Bangalore had to have a leg amputated. As he lived the process of adjusting to the trauma of that procedure, with the radical change in his lifestyle which it implies, the community worked to adapt their life to the needs of Ravi. Katharine, the community leader, explains that when Ravi was coming home after many weeks in hospital:

> We chose the central room in the house, we had bought new sheets and curtains. Ravi's bedroom is a public room – people come to visit all the time; they sit and chat; we moved evening prayers into his room, the house meeting too. The day workers feel free to come in…and Ravi looks out of the window where he can see the others going to work. In fact three days after coming home he announced he too wanted to go to work…so we initiated an hour in the work program even if he was just sitting. Everyone knows what is happening and has taken responsibility…yes there is some jealousy but in the main people want to be carers… We have been faithful to the small things – the dignity of his dress, the beauty of his room with flowers and personal possessions. (Hall 2006)

Chris, who is one of the younger members of the community, describes his experience:

> This year has been a full one with us all living the hospital-journey with Ravi. We prayed every night and visited him in hospital, and believed twice he was going to die…but he is home with us again. I like to help nurse him and have developed a strong friendship with him full of humour as I will not let him be sad over the fact he has lost one leg. I tease and play with him and sometimes sit with him while he sleeps or is sad. I try to encourage him to enjoy life. (Scott 2006)

Recognising that the person may need to move/collaboration with professionals in the medical and disability sectors

In order to ensure the best standards of care and support for community members, we need to work with professional people in the disability and medical fields. Sometimes it becomes clear that our community home is no longer the most appropriate setting in which to provide the care the person needs. At the same time we remain the primary point of reference for the person, along with family members. Depending on the nature of the disabling condition, the community member may need assistance in communicating needs or simple personal information. Medical professionals may have limited experience in working with people with intellectual disability. So we need to form good working partnerships.

Given the nature of our commitment to the person this will often imply organizing ourselves and the family and friends of the person to be with the person 24 hours a day, especially in hospital settings where things can change rapidly. The person needs to feel supported and information needs to be communicated accurately. Katharine describes the experience of being in the hospital with Ravi and of having to have him moved to different wards:

> Each move save the last one seemed to signify that we were not leaving and that the longed for healing was not happening... Each new move, each new difficulty in Ravi's condition was a process of stripping... There was the need to be intelligent and understand; to be able to obtain information from the doctors so that you did not feel like a piece of meat – examined but not related to... I railed with the nurses that they were not to DO to him without telling him before, even if he was semi-conscious. I tried to avoid the third person conversations about him but over him – BUT it happened. I struggled to maintain a dignity and a humanity. I insisted on shaving him every day and bathing him every day... I set up our own routine within the hospital patterns... We sang songs and said our prayers every morning and evening regardless of who was listening. I tried very hard never to leave him unaccompanied. I felt it was important to have the familiar close by so I brought in his pictures and I showed him these daily even when I had no response. I told him all my sorrows and hopes; told him news of the community and we phoned people and the community faithfully visited. (Hall 2006)

Almost without exception we hear from health-care professionals that they have never known a person with intellectual disability to be so supported in a hospital or hospice setting. We discover that our way of being with the person becomes educative for others involved in the provision of care.

Recognizing that loss and pain present opportunities for personal transformation

The community of Beni-Abbes in Hobart last year journeyed with one of their long-term members who had Alzheimer's disease. I was deeply moved to read the following reflection from the person who is responsible for the home where Ann lives:

> I had thought that this journey together would be all about minimising pain and suffering – all about loss – but to my continual surprise and delight, as time goes on, we're discovering that it's also about experiencing new ways to love and be loved. There is something incredibly humbling and illuminating about needing to reintroduce yourself to Ann on a day that she struggles to remember who you are. I had thought that this process would be terribly painful, but instead have found that in reality it is somehow freeing to be allowed to reintroduce myself to Ann, who I have known for about eighteen years. It gives us a unique opportunity to renew our relationship on a daily basis, whilst relaxing in the familiarity of our years together. As a result of this, a wonderful combination of the excitement of a new relationship with the comfort of an old friend is created, where new memories and old memories walk hand in hand. (Treanor and Vincent 2006, pp.177–78)

Cindy Treanor is a gifted musician who has written a song about her journey with Ann. It's called 'The Rollercoaster Ride', and one of the verses says

> You've helped me to see things I'd hidden away
> It's awakened in me
> Things no words can convey
> Will you journey with me, may I journey with you
> What surprises are in store?

The refrain is:

> So take your seat for the rollercoaster ride
> The highs and lows will make you cry
> Can I embrace my rollercoaster ride?
> It lets me know that I'm alive

and in the last refrain:

> Help me embrace your rollercoaster ride
> To live until we say goodbye.

A last word from Katharine in Bangalore:

> Ravi supported us all – the day I told him he was to die he stretched out his hand and stroked my head. Later on the ward, when I had just been told he had blood clotting on the brain and I was crying uncontrollably and trying to explain to him what that might mean for him, he did the same thing. Ravi was there for me in all my grief and loss and powerlessness... In the hospital many people asked me, 'Why are you here? Why do you stay with him?' My simple answer was, 'He is my brother'. One young intern asked me why I stayed with mentally handicapped people, why with Ravi when he never talked to me, never responded. I told him I was awaiting Ravi's smile which was worth so much...that I was awaiting the squeeze of my hand. Eventually I was forced to answer the question seriously for myself – why? I knew the answer quickly, 'because he gives me joy'...and that was amidst the discomfort, loneliness, anxiety, fear, pain, loss...yes, I knew joy. (Hall 2006)

Conclusion

The spirituality of L'Arche invites us to build relationships of friendship and mutuality, of forgiveness and celebration. It grounds us in an acceptance of the reality of human limitation and vulnerability. It teaches us that we do not need to be scandalized by our own needs, or weakness. With their capacity for directness, wonderment and compassion, people with intellectual disabilities become our greatest teachers, calling us to live authentically in relationship with one another.

In choosing to build lifelong relationships, we share the journey of growing older together and living the death of some of our friends. We have discovered our need to develop new competencies, to work with agencies and professional people in order to receive the support we need as well as to communicate the learning we have acquired. Over the years we are more deeply convinced that people with an intellectual disability have a place at the heart of the human family. Our challenge is to support them to offer their gifts, to live the fullness of their lives, and in that process we will all be enriched and transformed.

CHAPTER 6

Better Dead than Disabled?
When Ethics and Disability Meet:
A Narrative of Ageing,
Loss and Exclusion

Christopher Newell

I was tremendously proud of myself. After months of being in hospital and unable to attend the cathedral church within which I had been ministering for nine years, I was finally making it back to my church. Gulping the massive cocktail of drugs that made it possible for me to go in that morning, I ruefully reflected on all of the challenges associated with opioid drugs and the joys of wandering around feeling as if half of your brain has been removed due to the impact of morphine-type drugs. It was a moment of triumph. I had almost died and was literally back from the dead.

Yet when I arrived at my cathedral church I realized that I was not back from the dead and indeed that I was a part of the living dead. In retrospect I realized that the moment I reached the vestry I should have turned around and gone away. I found my robes strewn in the back of a vestry cupboard, trampled upon, dirty. There were to be no public words of welcome to me in the service, no giving thanks that I had returned despite almost dying. And after almost ten years of ministry at the cathedral I learned my true value. After years of sitting in a particular clergy pew in the cathedral I found that not only my place but also my role had been replaced by someone recently deaconed. 'You left us with a big gap, you know' she informed me as she bustled by. I found a small dusty corner in the cathedral to perch in, one eschewed by all others. There is a profound sense in which I learned that was my place, as someone ageing with disability.

Meanings found in disability and narrative

In this chapter I draw upon the insights of such exclusion to explore my experience of ageing with disability and the ethics to be found in the un-exceptional. As someone who has lived with disability all my life, I now realize that my traumatic admission to hospital was actually as a consequence of ageing with disability. The impossible that I had asked my body to do for so many years had finally given way in a screaming heap of spinal pain. As I sat in a Eucharist dedicated to the celebration of life, I wished that people had had the honesty to spit on me in the vestry as they passed me by rapidly. I wished that I really had died.

Looking back on it now I can but reflect ruefully on how I really had done the impossible, years ago in becoming an Anglican priest with disability when it was unthinkable in Australian society for people with disability to do this. (For an exploration see Goggin and Newell 2005; Newell and Calder 2004.)

Yet in this chapter I do more than reflect on the significance of the awful moment of reckoning. I also look at the transformation that has occurred recently, providing a happy ending to what started as an appalling state of exclusion.

Grief, loss and attitudes

There is no doubt that grief and loss figure prominently in my story. There is a raw wound which I have deliberately not covered. It is reproduced as originally written. This grief and loss was associated with further deterioration of my body leading to months in hospital over Christmas and a continuing process of rehabilitation, which continues today. A struggle with loss – when I thought I had already done the struggle with loss on a variety of other occasions as a person with lifelong disability. I recognized all of the symptoms – I even did all I could to avoid writing this.

Indeed I had looked up many books on ageing, encountering some resources as they relate to people with intellectual disability. It was safer to think about it happening to them. It is safer when we speak about the other rather than recognizing ageing and disability and further impairment happening to me. One volume in particular summed up many of the issues. Herr and Weber's 1999 collection *Aging, Rights, and Quality of Life: Prospects for Older People with Developmental Disabilities* I found to be an excellent secular resource. International authorities on ageing with regard to developmental disability explore important issues for this often forgotten population grouping. Much of it resonated with me as someone with other impairments who has also struggled with the challenge to my intellect associated with pain and drug therapy.

Herr and Weber's excellent resource covers such areas as principles of good practice, human rights, self-determination, managed care, developments in public policy, models for appropriate support, quality of life and the related quality standards, and legal and financial considerations. It is made all the more useful by the comprehensive research-base which is apparent, as well as the use of case studies. The ageing of adults with all types of disabilities is an important issue which has not necessarily received the intellectual energy that it should. This collection helpfully combines academic and practical considerations, making it a useful book for anyone who is concerned to improve the quality of life of older people with developmental disability.

Yet in reviewing that book and the literature in general, I became aware of something very significant: the lack of anything to do with the spiritual care or dimensions of people with disability; the failure to speak about ethical issues beyond the tried and empty 'autonomy rules OK'. I seek to address this in this chapter.

All of these factors combine with all the other aspects of loss associated with further onset of disability and in my case wondering if I would ever get back to a valued social position as Associate Professor at the University of Tasmania. We can certainly see evidence in my narrative of a continuing massive struggle with new levels of impairment, to keep going in socially valued roles: for example, in my role as an academic, to catch up with all of the articles that I should have written and whose deadlines I have missed. Having lived with disability all my life I thought I was well adapted. I had a lot to learn.

In all of this, attitudes play an important role. For me there is my own attitude as I have struggled with feelings of not only exclusion but also failure. In my experience, many of us with lifelong disability experience feelings of inadequacy when we cannot do the impossible any more and when the impossible catches up with us. This is compounded by the fact that often our bodies age quickly and earlier than social norms require. As a mentor of mine with disability who has also been through this said to me recently, 'We simply wear out.'

Within my academic writing I have critiqued dominant approaches to disability (Goggin and Newell 2005). Yet I found myself adopting these in my grief. Some of these dominant social attitudes may be summed up as:

Better off dead than disabled.

Thank God I don't have a disability.

Disability is about the other, rather than the us.

The irony is that these are the very values and stated ethics that most faith communities eschew. Yet they emerge in so much of the lived ethics of faith communities, and in my experience are revealed every day in the life of the church.

Likewise they are revealed in the euthanasia debate, as secular society makes its values very clear with persistent pushes for assisted suicide or what I prefer to name as medical killing (Newell 1996, 2000). Advocates for euthanasia explicitly avoid tackling the profound difficulties associated with such legislation, for those of us who are the living dead – people with a variety of disabilities. People who have never experienced living with disability are deeply distressed at the prospect of living with impairment and see medically assisted suicide as a logical option, the sanitary cure for that deeply unacceptable state – disability.[1]

Identity and the meta-narrative of disability

In all of this, the pervasiveness of the meta-narratives of disability is all-important. We are constituted by discourses and practices. Sadly much theological practice by churches and faith communities is based upon how negative disability, ageing with disability and the journey of impairment really is. My experience of further marginalization fits within such powerful accounts of reality and identity. As the noted narrative theorist Hilde Lindemann Nelson notes,

> How freely we can exercise our moral agency is contingent on a number of things. Most broadly, it depends on the form of life we inhabit: the niche we occupy in our particular society; the practices and institutions within the society that set the possibilities for the courses of action that are open to us; the material, cultural, and imaginative resources at our disposal; the constraints arising from the moral flaws within our roles and relationships; the shared moral understandings that render our actions intelligible to those around us. More specifically, the extent to which our moral agency is free or constrained is determined by our own – and others' – conception of who we are. (Nelson 2001, p.xi)

There can be little doubt these issues of 'who are we?' are ones we all face in the journey of life – something we inevitably have to confront no matter how powerful or rich we are. We find disability and ageing with disability as negative, in part because of the meta-narratives which tell us that impairment is negative rather than a way of encountering new rich dimensions of life, no matter how painful loss can be.

Accordingly I would suggest that the biggest problems I face are associated with very narrow attitudes and norms. No wonder ageing with disability is challenging.

Theological ethics in deeds

One of the continuing problems is that very few of us in churches, or faith communities in general, practice really good theological reflection. In particular, how well do we really explore what our lived values really say about ethics? Instead, we practise an account of ethics that does suggest 'better off dead than disabled' despite our pious statements to the contrary. We practise some very superficial accounts of faith which confirm our fears and prejudices. And yes, I realize that I am complicit in this, as I embrace the very dominant social values I critique.

Indeed, in writing this chapter I couldn't help reflecting on how the attitudes in theology that I encountered in my story of exclusion were to a significant extent a reflection of values contained within the leadership of the church in its espoused theology. I have been publishing on disability and theology for 15 years now, as well as speaking about it, and have even written reports at national level. Yet the power relations which disable continue. I would dare to suggest there are vested interests in keeping disability as other, second rate, pitiful. After all that is a key opportunity for church leaders to show their compassion as they bravely shake hands with the disabled, rush off to wash their hands hurriedly and then apply for a Bravery Medal.

A healthy church?

Related to this I would suggest that the situation is getting worse with managerial and simplistic and fundamentalist approaches to the so-called problems of the church. Bishops and church leaders are chosen for their managerial attributes and easy solutions.

For some years now some of us with disabilities have had significant problems with a document released by the Anglican Bishop of Tasmania, John Harrower, which argues for the importance of a 'healthy Church... transforming life'.[2] The jingoistic emphasis upon being healthy shows little regard for all of those critiques of functionalist accounts of the body I encountered way back in first-year Sociology. Instead such theology profoundly teaches those of us with bodies not deemed to be healthy, how unhealthy and ultimately unacceptable we are within faith communities. For all the attraction of simple solutions, I have come to realize how, in Australian churches that are increasingly struggling with declining numbers and no morale, such jingoistic simple solutions are extremely good at defining moral communities and shunning those who seem ultimately to contaminate the church.

At the same time I experienced the denial of my vocation as a priest with all that entails. I came to realize that even a retired elderly person is preferable to a person with disability, provided that person has a form of healthy ageing and does not display weakness or a lack of energy. In dominant accounts of the ethics of faith communities, such values are eschewed as the dignity (inherent worth) of all people is affirmed. Yet in our lived ethics, too often we are not allowed to be weak and there is no ministry to be found in presence or weakness.

These are accounts of theology – or rather superficial piety – which confirm our prejudices. Ultimately of course, when those peddling such models eventually become disabled, or age with disability, they have the opportunity to experience this for themselves, especially when they move beyond having power to powerlessness. Is it any wonder that we know we are better off dead than disabled?

Narrating and confirming otherness

I am reminded of the work of disabled American theologian, the late Bill Williams, who writes in this way about the creation of otherness:

> I have told you about my special ailments, whined a bit. But now you need to know something. I am not terribly unique. There are plenty of folks whose *principal wound* – the point of triage – is not the church's preoccupations, but an inability to accept the way they were made. This inability feels like an unending condemnation, an especially singular punishment for reasons undisclosed.

> For some it is a physical defect;
> Or having the wrong kind of 'subhuman' skin or shape to the eyes;
> Or being 'ugly' in a world that worships perfection;
> Or giving birth to a child with defects;
> Or being barren or sterile in a world that deifies parenthood;
> Or growing up in a sect that glorified shame;
> Or having the wrong gender or sexuality in a place that calls you inadequate or evil;
> Or having parents who crushed body and soul;
> Or being pushed to 'excel' in a way that said *never good enough*;
> Or being dyslexic; or having a short attention span; or possessing mechanical

intelligence in a school system that only recognizes agile, literate minds;
Or being freakishly smart;
Or being as Jewish as Christ in an aggressively Christian nation;
Or just being human. In some circles, that's bad enough.

The particulars of my experience are unique; but I am certainly not alone. In fact, and I admit, this might be the buy-a-van-and-see-all-the-vans-on-the-road effect, when I look around, I have this awful feeling that we may be the *majority*. (Williams 1998, pp.115–16)

The narration of the appalling nature of ageing and disability is also practised in secular society, played out on the front pages of newspapers we read. The promise of biotech cures for disability and ageing, provided we legislate cloning or fund enough science, means we often fund and legislate without really reflecting critically on the vested interests involved in narrating disability and ageing in this way of pathology and charity (Goggin and Newell 2004).

Indeed I want to suggest that much of the church's work in so-called 'safe ministry' reinforces the marginalization of the others towards which we must be safe. In the secular health literature about safety and quality at least we have started counting some of the adverse events. It is so sad that we have not explored what safety and quality in faith communities look like from the perspective of the poor and oppressed. After all I think there is a clear biblical precedent. We need an account of safety and quality which sees as vital knowledge the narratives of the displaced, diseased other, seeking to correct and lift up the oppressed. Dare I suggest reclaiming leadership for those we know to be other?

Brokenness and relationships

As horrible and terrible as my recent journey had been, such appalling 'character development' actually made me even better as a priest and person. Bill Williams says it so well for me:

If we disappear from your sight, it may be because our courage failed. We decided not to burden you, and ourselves, with our presence.

But I've been with people who are not made anxious by my brokenness, and I've seen the difference. It is, in fact, the best definition of ministry I have ever heard; I nearly wept when I heard it, it so defined what I needed. Engrave this upon your forehead, if you would wish to do good:

Ministry is a non-anxious presence

You can tell such grace by its care, by its attentive ear, by its pace. When it reaches out to heal you, it is to give relief to you, not itself – and when it prays with you, it lets you declare your own burdens, rather than declaring what it finds burdensome about you. (Williams 1998, pp.32–3)

In all of this, relationships are central. It is relationships that help people to know that they are valued – or horribly devalued, worthy of death. Ultimately it is relationships that form our attitudes and indeed assist with ethical decisions such as resources allocation. Ageing with disability raises significant issues on whether or not we can actually discern and find ministry in the context of ultimate weakness, frailty and death.

Recently I also started publishing out of my experiences of the valley of the shadow of death in a hospital bed (Newell 2006): compelling narrative and theology, my friends tell me, yet also raising important questions: How can we as a church affirm that broken people have something profound and sacred to offer as leaders in exploring and discovering the good and sacred life? Further, such writings are indicative of a weakness that I cannot overcome – and why should I feel the need to do so?

Relationships have also meant that I have struggled with an appropriate ending to this chapter, because, rather than a sad and bitter ending, I have recently found hope and affirmation that in my brokenness there is much I have to offer. It all stems from the ministry of the current Dean of St David's Cathedral, Dr Lindsay Stoddart, who has found a central place for me. Indeed I recently was given a stall and a position as Canon Theologian at St David's Cathedral, a valued position within the Anglican tradition. I remember well how he visited me in hospital. We talked for a long time and the handshake at the end was indicative of a hand of friendship where I was drawn back into a valued place in the very community within which I felt I had no place. The fact that I am not healthy is an asset and not a liability.

I knew there was no place left for me in my faith community. I now know the embrace of a valued role. Ageing with disability has been reconceptualized by a colleague who shares my understanding of brokenness.

Conclusion: claiming the sacred

Ultimately the horrible times I have discussed in this chapter, including the marginalization within the church, are part of a sacred journey, a getting of wisdom. As Frederic and Mary Ann Brussat argue,

Life is a sacred adventure. Every day we encounter signs that point to the active presence of Spirit in the world around us. Spiritual literacy is the ability to read the signs written in the texts of our own experiences. Whether viewed as a gift from God or a skill to be cultivated, this facility enables us to discern and decipher a world full of meaning.

Spiritual literacy is practised in all the world's wisdom traditions. Medieval Catholic monks called it 'reading the book of the world'. Muslims suggest that everything that happens outside and inside us is a letter to be read. Native Americans find their way through the wilderness by 'reading sign'. From ancient times to today, spiritually literate people have been able to locate within their daily life, points of connection with the sacred. (Brussat and Brussat 1996, p.15)

If there is one thing almost as certain as death and taxes, it is that if we live long enough then we will almost inevitably have to face up to disability. For, as we age, we often acquire impairments. For those of us born with disability or impairment acquired earlier in life, ageing often brings the joys associated with further challenges to function, and the opportunity to be the latest statistic labelled as having a syndrome. In a death- and disability-denying society, disability becomes the living death for those who acquire impairment as they age. This situation is further compounded by the focus of society, informed by medical and charitable discourses about disability, or miracle cures. As we have seen, disability is constructed as the private tragedy and responsibility of the individual. Euthanasia and resources allocation debates may be seen as symptoms of broader ethical issues, untackled in the public arena. In all of these we can see that there is a deep spiritual dimension to the dominant knowledge we have of ageing and of acquiring disability in later life. Rather than being inherently negative, we may find essential human dimensions and depth associated with that which we fear most deeply, ageing and disability.

Right relationships not only are important in nurturing those of us with disability but also allow those of us with disability to nurture. Ultimately faith and secular communities are constantly engaged in addressing and answering the question 'better dead than disabled?' All around the world church leaders talk piously of the importance of healthy churches and the easy solutions to life provided you follow their ten-point plan. I can but suggest that life is sacred not despite disability, but also through the woundedness we all share as persons.

Notes

1 This is reflected in a recent 'Four Corners' ABC TV programme in Australia, which documented the situation of older Australians who seek euthanasia if they acquire disability as they age. See www.abc.net.au/4corners/content/2007/s1914206.htm.

2 See www.anglicantas.org.au/resources/index.html.

CHAPTER 7

Disabled or Enabled: Ethical and Theological Issues for Dementia Care

Rosalie Hudson

By 2040 there will be over 80 million people with dementia worldwide, increasing at the rate of one every seven seconds (Alzheimer's Disease International 2006, p.1). In Australia by 2016 dementia will become the largest cause of disability burden after depression, continuing to outpace other chronic illnesses (Alzheimer's Australia 2003, p.iv). Does this impose an intolerable burden on service providers, or does it provide unprecedented opportunities, particularly for those responsible for pastoral care? This chapter will suggest how spirituality, personhood and ethics are to be understood theologically, using examples to ground these concepts in contemporary best practice dementia care. Language will be shown as an important ethical and theological indicator, with the power to *dis*able or to *en*able. An emphasis on the burden and dependency associated with dementia will be shown to reflect the predominant contemporary culture of individualism rather than a Christian understanding of persons in community. Throughout the chapter the emphasis is on relationships, indicating the richness and freedom that comes from understanding ourselves not as individual monads but as persons in relationship or in community with each other. In conclusion, a response is offered from a hypothetical person with dementia who has been enabled in the face of this profoundly disabling illness.

Language for dementia

What language do we use to describe a person with dementia? Is the language enabling or disabling? Commonly used *dis*abling descriptions include 'she's away with the fairies', 'all the lights are out and there's nobody home', 'upstairs

81

is vacant', 'the person is no longer there, he's just a shell'. This kind of disabling language, together with labels such as 'sufferers' or 'victims', implies a state of utter helplessness and hopelessness. 'This not only strips people of their dignity and self-esteem, it reinforces inaccurate stereotypes and heightens the fear and stigma surrounding dementia' (Alzheimer's Australia 2004, p.1).

When the nature of dementia is misunderstood, terms such as 'dementing' and 'demented' are often used. These terms suggest a defining characteristic; the person is labelled and objectified, reinforcing the stereotype, the fear and the stigma of dementia. Understanding dementia as an umbrella term that covers a wide and complex group of illnesses enables a more personalized approach. Bryden, speaking from personal experience, says: 'Please don't call us "dementing" – we are still people separate from our disease, we just have a disease of the brain. If I had cancer you would not refer to me as "cancerous", would you' (Bryden 2005, p.141). Similarly disabling, not only for one person with dementia but for a group of people, is the stereotypical and dehumanizing term 'the dementias'. As Bryden suggests, people with cancer are not referred to as 'the cancers'.

When a person is described as 'demented' the condition is placed before the person rather than the other way round, a process Kitwood identifies as 'malignant social psychology' (Kitwood 1997, pp.46–7). The intent is not malicious; however, the categorization is dehumanizing. 'People with dementia are individuals first and the condition should not be regarded or referred to as the defining aspect of their life' (Alzheimer's Australia 2004, p.4). Language is a powerful tool that can disable or enable, particularly in the context of dementia care. Health professionals and the wider community are therefore being encouraged to replace demeaning terms and bureaucratic jargon with a more personalized and empowering language. This is not to diminish the profoundly disabling consequences of dementia. However, while the experience of dementia can be heartbreaking, tragic, devastating, terrible, painful, distressing and debilitating, it need not be hopeless, unbearable or impossible (Alzheimer's Australia 2004, p.5). The emphasis of this chapter is on adopting a more thoughtful and considered approach to dementia care, conveyed in particular by our language and by our attitudes to burden and disability.

The burden of disability

'Mum never wanted to be a burden', says the distraught daughter at the bedside. Her mother is in the advanced stages of dementia and decisions need to be made about treatment interventions. 'Shoot me if I ever get like that!' says the frustrated nurse to her colleagues. The notion of burden is having a profound influence on end-of-life decision-making; from those on the one hand who clearly articulate their advance care directives, to those on the other hand who call for physician-assisted suicide rather than contemplate dying with dementia. There is no question about the extent of disability and dependency accompanying advanced dementia and we can understand the dilemma and heartache this causes families and carers. Inevitably, onlookers will imagine themselves in this situation and contemplate their response. The challenge for service providers is: how can they *en*able people with dementia and their family carers to live hopefully while experiencing the *dis*abling manifestations of dementia?

Contemporary culture, with its emphasis on vibrant youth and wrinkle-free, healthy ageing, does not look kindly on burden, disability, dependency or suffering. Hauerwas says:

> We especially fear, if not dislike, those whose suffering is the kind for which we can do nothing. They are not self-sufficient, they are not self-possessed, they are in need. Even more, they do not evidence the proper shame for being so... It is almost as if they have been given a natural grace to be free from the regret most of us feel for our neediness... We do not like to be reminded of the limits of our power, and we do not like those who remind us. (Hauerwas 1986, p.176)

Furthermore, claims Hauerwas, when suffering is perceived only in a negative sense, there seems to be no alternative to eradicating it. The Christian concept of suffering is paradoxical; while it is an inevitable part of human existence we are urged to do all in our power to eliminate suffering wherever we can. To accept the inevitability of suffering is not to suggest that suffering should be sought, glorified, idealized or merely accepted for its own sake. It is to suggest, however, that many people experience both the pain of suffering and the benefits of enduring the suffering for which there is no solution. This endurance is made bearable, of course, when others are willing to stand alongside those who are suffering, offering them compassion and practical support. There is, however, a strange deduction made by a society that sees euthanasia as the most 'compassionate' solution in relation to dementia or other life-threatening disease. 'It seems odd that in the name of eliminating suffering, we eliminate the sufferer' (Hauerwas 1986, p.24).

It is impossible to calculate or quantify the suffering experienced by a person with dementia, so attention is drawn again to the arbitrary and disabling use of the term 'dementia sufferers'. Because each person with dementia is unique we ought not make assumptions such as 'people with dementia don't suffer' or 'all people with dementia experience an enormously high level of suffering'. Best practice dementia care relies, for example, on readily available guidelines for pain management and symptom control, using the principles of impeccable assessment (Commonwealth of Australia 2006, pp.61–8). Based on the evidence that many people in the advanced stage of dementia experience symptoms similar to those in the last stage of cancer, the onus is on service providers to ensure appropriate symptom assessment and intervention is available to relieve suffering wherever possible. Contemporary research is also uncovering the magnitude of suffering and burden experienced by family members and friends caring for people with dementia (Goldsmith 2004), indicating the increasing need for the church's pastoral care.

However, even in the midst of a profoundly saddening and disturbing experience of living with dementia, both informal and formal carers attest to experiences of humour, joy and surprise. Killick and Allan (2001) tell many delightful stories to exemplify the range of responses from people with dementia, particularly when the principles of thoughtful and sensitive communication are practised. The language of burden, therefore, needs to acknowledge ambivalence; all situations are not necessarily hope-less and the experience can change from moment to moment. The language of burden needs also to acknowledge the incalculable presence of love experienced by many people with dementia and their carers. This adds a fresh ingredient to the concept of burden, as Meilaender thoughtfully observes. Contemplating the use of advance directives in the context of dementia or other debilitating illness, Meilaender decides he does want to be a burden to his wife.

> I hope, therefore, that I will have the good sense to empower my wife, while she is able, to make such decisions for me... No doubt this will be a burden to her. No doubt she will bear the burden better than I would. No doubt it will be only the last in a long history of burdens she has borne for me. But then, mystery and continuous miracle that it is, she loves me. And because she does, I must of course be a burden to her. (Meilaender 1991, p.14)

Personhood and spirituality

Can a renewed understanding of 'burden' influence our care of people with dementia? How does a theological understanding of personhood help us to provide pastoral care for people who no longer know their own name? What does it mean for people with dementia to know they are made in the image of God when they can no longer recognize their own image in a mirror? What does the body language of love convey when words elicit no response?

Personhood and spirituality, understood from the perspective of Christian theology, are first and foremost *relational* terms and are therefore *enabling*. Personhood is a communal reality made possible by the gracious and deeply personal Trinitarian call of God. God the Father, in love and freedom for the world, sends the Son to enact that love, calling us all, by the power of the Spirit, to our true humanity. On this understanding, it is God's faithfulness to us that is more important than our understanding or our measure of *our* faithfulness to God. The Psalmist says:

> How precious to me are *thy* [emphasis added] thoughts, O God, how vast is the sum of them! If I should count them, they are more in number than the sand: when I awake, I am still with thee. (Psalm 139:17–18, KJV)

Waking or sleeping, conscious or unconscious, even in Sheol, the place of forgetfulness and dust, God remembers us. This is surely a welcome, enabling word of hope for those unable to charter alone the smallest journey from bed to bathroom (Hudson 2004b).

God *is*, as three persons, always and only *in relationship*, not for God's self-satisfaction or to confront us with an impenetrable geometric conundrum, but *for our sake*, to enable us to be in relationship with God and each other. The essence of the triune relationships is on their *interrelatedness* or their *co-dependency*: each needs the other to enable the full expression of God's love to be realized. An ancient Greek term for this interrelationship is perichoresis, literally meaning 'to dance around' (LaCugna 1991, p.271). The concept of dancing has been widely used in art and literature to depict the reality of our final journey towards death. Bryden has taken this theme and applied it to her experience of living with dementia in order to emphasize the importance of keeping in step with one's partner (Bryden 2005). The perichoretic relationships in the Holy Trinity reveal the true nature of love: it is totally personal, totally mutual, and totally reciprocal. Furthermore, when it is translated into human relationships, no person is excluded. This means a person with dementia is not 'less whole' than others, for personhood is not lost when cognitive powers fail (Hudson 2004a, p.95). Trinitarian theology shows that love can only flourish when persons live in relationship; interdependency is the key.

This interdependence is not built on common characteristics, emotional magnetism or shared philosophical values. Nor is it built on physical capacity or intellectual prowess. Furthermore, this relationship is not predicated on our potential – what we hope to become by sheer effort and striving. Given these criteria, people with dementia would not be included. The mystery and the freedom of the triune relationships is in the unqualified, undeserved love in which we are recognized for who we are and *as we are now*. That is indeed good news for those who have lost the capacity to recognize who and what they are, or even to demonstrate love in return. This does not give any of us cause for self-satisfaction, for it does not negate our call to holiness and perfection and for obedient discipleship. The good news is that we are not solely dependent on our own individual capacity; within the Body of Christ each member is dependent on the others.

On this understanding, we are prompted to question the measure we use to determine the capacity of a person with dementia. 'Don't worry about visiting', we advise relatives, 'she doesn't know who you are'. This comment arises from the cultural presupposition that individuals are self-contained, with no need of others, and that the person with dementia has such a poor quality of life that relationships are meaningless. MacKinlay's research shows, however, that 'relationship is almost synonymous with meaning for people with dementia' (MacKinlay 2006a, p.179). Service providers who understand the language of relationship will encourage family members to continue visiting; as a sign of human solidarity and a sign of the vulnerability and interdependency that characterizes all our lives. Furthermore, none of us can be sure what awareness the person with dementia retains. There is sufficient evidence from the experience of many people to show that, in sometimes rare moments of lucidity, the person is far more 'aware' than we previously thought. The language of relationship also encourages service providers, and particularly pastoral carers, to offer sensitive and thoughtful support to those family carers who find visiting a strain.

Relationship is the essence of spirituality. The concept of spirituality as a rationally constructed private retreat into one's inner being is the prevailing theme of our 'hypercognitive' Western culture. That does not provide, however, a meaningful response to the person who is losing cognition. Our relentless dependence on the cosy combination of words and works allows us little headway into the world of dementia. Those of us familiar with the demands of Clinical Pastoral Education would know that the person with end stage dementia does not make a compelling case study for the ubiquitous *verbatim*. How then do we engage in pastoral care in the absence of meaningful conversation, particularly when the person is unable to distinguish the chaplain from the cook? Another way must be found unless we are to join those who believe people with dementia are non-persons 'already in the house of the dead' (Post 1995, pp.18–9).

Perhaps the person with dementia – freed from all pretension, totally incapable of spiritual self-examination – might be an icon of God's grace to us? Here, we stumble across our own incapacity to live communally, especially with those disabled in body or mind. We prefer, even in our churches, to commune and harmonize with those of like mind, constructing physical and other more subtle barriers for those who are different. Here again, we are prone to reflect the values of the culture rather than the counter-cultural claims of the Christian Gospel.

In the divine dance of Trinitarian love we are welcomed as partners; we are drawn into the fellowship of Father, Son and Spirit, even when we have forgotten the steps. In our cultural milieu where Descartes' dictum 'I think, therefore I am' rules our political, economic and organizational processes, there is no place for the person with declining rational capacity. How then can we enable one another pastorally in the context of ageing and disability? Can we chart a spiritual course of pastoral care for people with dementia? Perhaps we start by recognizing the illusions that frame our thoughts and actions. We live by an illusion that we can be totally free, independent individuals, capable of plotting our own steps on our own private spiritual journey. 'This is *my* life, *my* journey, *my* spiritual quest', we say, 'and you have no *right* to invade my private space'. For Lewis, realities of infirmity, disability and mortality expose this illusion:

> The truth, which humanity at large is busy denying, is that we all have a *proper* inability to be persons alone, and need others to be our own, free selves. Such freedom entails the risk that others will try to own – or disown – us… And when we banish the dependent to a sub-world of their own, the guilt and fear they expose in us are proof enough that they belong with us in ours. (Lewis 1982, p.16)

Inquiry into the meaning of dementia, trying to explore the human everyday lived *experience* of dementia rather than its objectifying, defining characteristics, reminds us of our own frailty. When we consider the dependent nature of dementia we are prompted to ask ourselves which of us is *never* dependent on others. In the context of disability, we are prompted to ask ourselves which of us is *never* disabled in any way. From the moment of our conception we need someone to accompany us on this sometimes hazardous journey through life. At many stages on that journey we are dependent, for shorter or longer periods, on others. None of us has the capacity to live life on our own. When we regard people with dementia as intolerable burdens, or as those incapable of response, we rob them of the opportunity of relationships. If, on the other hand, we enjoy renewed confidence in the triune relationships of freely given love, we know (by faith rather than sight) that no person is excluded. If we were to secure for ourselves a 'place' in this dance of love we would be relying on our own estimation of worthiness and on this measurement others would be considered unworthy: a concept utterly opposed to Trinitarian love.

Taking this analogy further, if we exclude a person with dementia from any experience on the basis of our perception of their reality, we add to their disability. In contrast, when we *enable* a person with dementia to experience familiar people and places or to enjoy new opportunities, we engage in healing relationships. Bryden implores her readers not to deny her the pleasure of such experiences, even though she may not recall them five minutes later.

> As we become more emotional and less cognitive, it's the way you talk to us, not what you say, that we will remember. We know the feeling, but don't know the plot. Your smile, your laugh and your touch are what we will connect with. (Bryden 2005, p.138)

This is spirituality at work. It is instructive to note here that many writers are grappling with the contemporary meaning of spirituality; how it is to be understood, how it might be measured, and what assessment tools will provide a valid and reliable set of data for health professionals. Bryden, from within her own unique world of dementia, is a consummate teacher. She regards the smile, the laugh and the touch as indispensable keys to spirituality. 'We need love, comfort, attachment, inclusion, identity and occupation as our world around us becomes strange and our ability scrambled', she adds (p.144).

Within the constraints of this chapter it is not possible to draw out the implications of Bryden's comments for issues such as worship and pastoral care in residential aged care facilities and other settings. Questions are raised, however, as to whether some current practices actually further disable people with dementia by excluding them, rather than enabling them to experience spiritual nurture and growth. One poignant example relates to a conversation amongst carers about 'Jimmy' who was considered 'a lost soul'. Sacks takes up the story:

> 'Watch Jimmy in the chapel,' they said, 'and judge for yourself'. I did, and I was moved, profoundly moved and impressed, because I saw here an intensity and steadiness of attention and concentration that I had never seen before in him or conceived him capable of. I watched him kneel and take the Sacrament on his tongue, and could not doubt the fullness and totality of Communion, the perfect alignment of his spirit with the spirit of the Mass. Fully, intensely, quietly, in the quietude of absolute concentration and attention, he entered and partook of the Holy Communion. He was wholly held, absorbed, by a feeling. There was no forgetting, no Korsakov's then, nor did it seem possible or imaginable that there should be; for he was no longer at the mercy of a faulty and fallible mechanism – that of meaningless sequences and memory traces – but was absorbed in an act, an act of his whole being, which carried feeling and meaning in an organic continuity and unity, a continuity and unity so seamless it could not permit any break. (Sacks 1985, p.36)

Recalling the descriptions in the opening paragraph of this chapter, Sacks' story is a salutary reminder of the judgments we make when referring to a person as 'no longer there' or 'just an empty shell' or 'a lost soul'. This has particular implications for who is to be included, or excluded, in worship or other activities either in a nursing home or the local parish. In theological terms, we do violence to the Body of Christ if we exclude any person, particularly on the basis of their cognitive capacity, from participating in such communion.

Sacks' story also makes clear the inadequacy of empirical science for determining what constitutes personal being, so he adds:

> Perhaps there is a philosophical as well as a clinical lesson here: that in Korsakov's, or dementia, or other such catastrophes, however great the organic damage and human dissolution, there remains the undiminished possibility of reintegration by art, by communion, by touching the human spirit: and this can be preserved in what seems at first a hopeless state of neurological devastation. (Sacks 1985, pp.38–9)

Sacks' scientific background and his anthropological research provide fresh insights into the brain and our perception of cognitive incapacity. Through Sacks' lens we view the paradox of dementia. While it seems to our rational mind that the heart and soul of the person are 'lost', it may be that within the plaques and tangles of the brain the full human person emerges (Kimble 1990, p.32). While it seems that the person with dementia is inexorably becoming isolated in 'their own world', the person may 'emerge' when prompted by continuous, loving, faithful relationships. While it seems the person with dementia has no need for external stimuli ('he doesn't know where he is, so don't bother taking him on the bus') those very stimuli may be a means to fulfilling experiences.

Having suggested, by a very brief excursus into the Trinitarian theology of personhood and spirituality, that daily practice can be enhanced by relationships, it now remains to further unite theory and practice in an exploration of ethics at the end of life.

Ethics at the end of life

The spirit of this chapter is about contrasting *dis*abling relationships with *en*abling relationships and drawing out the implications for theological and spiritual reflection on practice. Rather than rehearsing all the end-of-life ethico-legal concepts readily available to health professionals, this section begins with a description of the final chapter in the life of one older person with dementia.

He is curled up in a little ball, right in the middle of the nursing home bed. Although he is tiny, never moving spontaneously, the safety rails are always raised. The only sign of his responsiveness is through his eyes, but everyone says 'He's demented; he can't communicate at all.'

He suffers from repetitive chin movements, which makes it terribly difficult to assist him with food and drink. He is often left unshaven. 'He's always been like that', says one carer, with mind-numbing presumption about his 88 pre-admission years. 'We don't get him up because he's more comfortable in bed', the nurses tell each other. His difficult, unfamiliar name suggests he is not Anglo-Saxon but no one knows for sure. Few of the staff can pronounce Demetrious Papadopolous so they've shortened his name to 'Poppa'.

He has no family and very few clothes or personal belongings. His care is often left until last. He receives no pastoral care because the 'religion box' is marked 'nil'. Now that he is dying, some of the nurses are concerned he may not be given as much attention as some of the other residents. Others say, 'If ever there was a case for euthanasia, this is it. Shoot me if I ever get like that!'

A new nurse unit manager was appointed, who had completed a course in person-centred dementia care. Carefully sifting through the fragmented notes she found that Mr Papadopolous had a considerable amount of money in the care of the State Trustees. Armed with this, and other important information including lack of interventions for several painful physical conditions, she called a brief meeting with the chaplain, the lifestyle coordinator and some of the nurses. She told them she was concerned Mr Papadopolous was not receiving the care he deserved. 'How can we get to know him so we can personalize his care?' she said. 'I notice his hygiene is often left until last, and I know the staff find him unattractive and difficult. Do we know what his spiritual needs are?' Together, a small team of committed carers focused on what was possible. Money was spent on his clothing, an electric shaver, a mobile water chair; the social worker who assessed him for admission was contacted. She provided the link for the local Greek Orthodox (GO) Church, and Mr Papadopolous' response had to be seen to be believed, when the priest in his familiar regalia came to his bedside.

Gradually, other staff came to see Mr Papadopolous as a person no less deserving of care than others who were more responsive. The regular chaplain coordinated the visits of the GO priest, making sure she also visited Mr Papadopolous whenever she could. Visitors to other residents in the shared room also began to greet Mr Papadopolous, even though his response was difficult to discern. A genuine transformation was taking place; ethical care was clearly interwoven with enabling Mr Papadopolous to enjoy the same quality of care as others. Slowly, and as a direct result of others modelling a different way of relating to Mr Papadopolous, attitudes changed. In particular, staff noticed the nurse unit manager going first to his bedside. She used positive, life-affirming, relational language when reporting at handover. 'I've found Mr Papadopolous will sometimes respond with his eyes when I speak gently to him, and now that we've commenced him on a low dose of morphine he's no longer resistive to care.' In the absence of speech Mr Papadopolous was given a voice.

Mahatma Gandhi has reminded us that the way we treat the 'last person' is a measure of our humanity. When the person with dementia is left until last, or regarded as unworthy of immediate attention, we may call to mind Nazi Germany where those with mental illness were considered unworthy of life. The Nazi analogy is also seen in its proximal reality, rather than its remoteness, when dementia is referred to as 'a living death' or when a person with dementia is referred to as 'no longer a person: she might as well be dead'. While we can understand the context of these responses and sympathize with the emotional turmoil that gives rise to them, a Christian understanding of personhood enables another way of thinking and speaking and acting.

In the Trinitarian model of relationships there is no hierarchy; each person is related to others not by their capacity to understand or respond but according to their unique image, made in the likeness of God. Rather than this 'measure' we prefer to make our own judgments about 'quality of life'. 'His quality of life is below zero, so let's not have any heroics!' This stance often results in less protection being given to those deemed undeserving. Sadly, this also often results in sub-optimal care. For example, 'basic nursing care' can be a 'rationale' for neglecting important issues such as pain management, spiritual, emotional and psychological care which may require complex, skilled interventions. These observations do not overlook the fact that there are many exceptional examples of creative, imaginative, person-centred dementia care, and increasing examples of a palliative approach being used to great effect for people dying in the advanced stages of dementia. However, more encouragement is needed to consider *enabling relationships* as one of the most urgent ethical issues of our time.

Reference has been made above to the increasingly helpful use of advance directives to ensure that ethical decision-making is in the best interests of the person who is dying. Ethical concentration should be on the needs of the person with dementia, not the needs of the family. Where a suitable, trusted person has been appointed 'proxy' in this matter, the issues are usually less complicated. However, serious ethical issues arise when no such person has been appointed, or when there is disagreement among family members about the treatment options. In residential aged care, as well as in other settings, the best course of action is considered to be a family meeting, attended also by the doctor, in which goals of care are explored until agreement is reached (Commonwealth of Australia 2006, p.57). In the absence of agreement a formal guardian may need to be appointed.

While particular ethical issues might be different in each situation, a common ethical response centres on open communication and trust. In a well-planned meeting, the form of questions to guide discussion is important. For example, rather than asking 'What would the person have wanted?' it might be more helpful to ask 'What is best for the person at this particular time in this particular situation?' Rather than trying to quantify quality of life, as implied by the question 'Is this person's life worth living any longer?', a more helpful question would be 'What can we do to enhance (or enable) the life that the person still has?' Subsequent discussion would include correct and reliable information for families, developing a plan of care based on contemporary evidence-based research and continually building a relationship of trust.

Enabling and disabling

If we are feeling rather daunted by the relatively recent changes in contemporary dementia care, if we are feeling that we have not adequately understood the issues of disabling and enabling relationships in the context of profound disability, then we are not alone. In his illuminating book *Dependent Rational Animals*, MacIntyre makes a correction to his earlier works in acknowledgment of his failure to adequately treat the subject of vulnerability and dependence on others. He claims that historically Western moral philosophy has also been negligent:

> From Plato to Moore and since there are usually, with some rare exceptions only passing references to human vulnerability and affliction and to the connections between them and our dependence on others... And when the ill, the injured and the otherwise disabled are presented in the pages of moral philosophy books, it is almost always exclusively as possible subjects of benevolence by moral agents who are themselves presented as though they were continuously rational, healthy and untroubled. So we are invited, when we do think of disability, to think of 'the disabled' as 'them', as other than 'us', as a separate class, not as ourselves as we have been, sometimes are now and may well be in the future. (MacIntyre 1999, pp.1–2)

Returning to the statistics quoted at the beginning of the chapter, it is unlikely that any of us will remain untouched, either personally or professionally, by the disabling aspects of dementia. MacIntyre urges us to avoid placing people with dementia in a separate world; rather, he encourages us to consider ourselves not apart from those with disabilities but as integrally related.

Conclusion

Is it humanly possible to be hope-*full* in a seemingly hope-less situation, to be an enabling influence in the presence of the disabling disease of dementia? I have tried in this chapter to convey, through a theological framework grounded in practice, a means of nurturing hope even in the most tragic situation. In conclusion, and prompted by the experience of Scott-Maxwell (Scott-Maxwell 1968, pp.75,138) I have painted a word picture of how this enabling might appear to a person with dementia.

Spending my last days on this journey, I am able to be myself; dancing a creative tango with all my carers. I am now in a place where my 'wandering' is not considered a problem, my idiosyncrasies are acknowledged and having 'a mind of my own' is not regarded as deviant behaviour. My variant moods also are no cause for blame or shame. Though dependent on others I am not left in isolation; my family and friends are welcomed as fellow travellers on this highway.

Here I need not fear abandonment; I will be cared for no matter how strange and muddled and directionless I may appear. On this road, my deepest spiritual yearnings are met through companionship, understanding and humour. Here I am known not only for what I am, but also for who I have been and who I may yet become.

CHAPTER 8

On Relationships Not Things: Exploring Disability and Spirituality

Lorna Hallahan

Introduction: the priority of belonging

Mark Thomsen, reflecting on the life and death of his small granddaughter, asserts that 'to be or to be human is first to belong' (2004, p.316). He argues that this belonging takes priority over thinking and doing. Drawing on two recent studies in disability and theology, this chapter argues that the 'belonging' of many people living with disability is threatened. It advances an understanding of disability as intersubjective. An understanding that shifts a sole focus on functional impairment towards a detailed analysis of social and intimate relationships, it builds a spacious foundation on which to develop engaged understandings of spirituality. This chapter also affirms spirituality as intersubjective – a crucial understanding for those who want to enrich the transformative potential of their work alongside ageing and disabled people. Invoking the concept of 'thin places', the chapter advocates an engaged, collective spirituality that gives voice and moral depth to a search for the humane, life-affirming heart and mind in contact with marginalized people. It offers some resources to develop a spirituality that seeks not simply to console but to challenge and empower. It sustains our hopes and our actions; gives energy and vitality to our attempts to belong to communities of support and solidarity; and breaks the bonds that place others beyond the scope of our moral concern.

Disability as intersubjective

Threatened belonging

From 2000 to 2003, I coordinated a project called 'Beyond the Ramp: The Work of Embrace', exploring disability and spirituality in order to empower people with impairments and their supporters, in their quest for embrace in the faith community of their choice. The project emerged from a national conference held in South Australia in 1998 which identified exclusion from faith communities as a major issue for people living with disability. Contemporaneously, I conducted doctoral studies in disability theory and Christian systematic theology (Hallahan 2005). This chapter combines findings from both investigations.

Beyond the Ramp worked with three large, well-established urban congregations of the Uniting Church of Australia and applied an action-research model using the strengths of the faith community as the major resources to bridge into identified areas of concern about the minimal participation of people living with disability at the heart of congregational life. The project produced strategies and resources applied within, in the participating congregations and in other interested faith communities. It was not an external-expert-driven approach, but was based on preferring to see that those who live within a community are best equipped to clarify their vision, identify strengths and resources, and truthfully name points where the community falls short of its best intentions. This implies initial attention to relationships, not structures.

The research analysed existing relationships with people with impairments and looked into congregational structures, attitudes and practices that inhibit or facilitate increased participation. It revealed that these three faith communities were not significantly different from other community organizations in Australian cities. Looking generally across the three congregations, people with impairments fell into three categories: first, a number of people with impairments – often but not always age-related– truly belong within the life and work of the congregation. There is a second, larger category of people with whom the relationships could only be described as formal and instrumental. These are people who are not bound by affiliation but by the desire to *do* something worthwhile in their lives. They often reported feelings of exclusion, not being welcome, being overlooked and uncomfortable in church activities. The final grouping comprised non-participant targets of outreach and mission. Analysed from this perspective, it is clear that many people with impairments experience disability primarily as a crisis in belonging.

These findings, while unsurprising, reflected a growing understanding among disability theorists that common-sense understandings of disability as organic impairment – a feature of bodies and minds, an attribute of an individual – are inadequate to respond to the complexity of life with disability. The social model, advocated within the sociological and political literature, distinguishes between the organic impairment, or condition, and disability as socially and politically constructed, saying 'there is no such thing as a disabled person, just a disabling society'. This position can also been seen as too dualistic or abstract and therefore limiting. So, alongside increasing evidence that people living with disability continue to experience high levels of marginalization and exclusion, I interpret this as an invitation to value everyday lived experience, quests for meaning and the individual's desire for connection and flourishing.

The force field of disability

Working with Henrietta Moore's (1994) model of intersubjectivity (a theory that argues that difference is created in the relationships we have, not in the bodies we have) Moore invites us to see that

> Experience is [thus] intersubjective and embodied; it is not individual and fixed, but irredeemably social. The experience of being a woman or being black or being Muslim can never be a singular one, and will always be dependent on a multiplicity of locations and positions that are constructed socially, that is intersubjectively. (p.3)

I find it helpful to think of a force field of disability based on the following five main elements:

- First, the difficult body in which we recognize and give due weight to our sharp moments of living with impairment, experiences of facing medical crises, of living with dread and fear, of not being able to make sense of the world around us and acknowledge that we must everyday face these difficulties and frailties.

- Second, a history of oppression and exclusion so graphically represented by the nineteenth-century 'crippleages' that still hold the horizon in our cities and the 'communitions' of the current day – mini-institutions lurking in our suburbs.

- Third, sociological circumstances, lived so often as exclusion and oppression – shaping our lives in the terrain of low expectations and discrimination, dealing with the forces of disablism. It is important to say something about the profile of relationships we see in the lives of Australians living with disability. Many people who self-identify as needing assistance to live with their impairments also describe daily lives passed almost exclusively in the company of family members and other intimate relationships. They have restricted access to the worlds of work, recreation and education, and travel only within a limited range from their homes. Their 'carers' are unpaid and their supports informal. At times this is a wonderful source of support and strength, and at times it is isolating and confronting for all those within the family. Then there are the lives of many people who continue to live almost exclusively outside intimate relationships – they only have contact with paid carers, they also have restricted access to their communities but may travel distances just to go to services or day activities. Where they have supports, these are always formal.

- Fourth, 'the secret places of the heart' – which is social worker Judith Lee's expression for the ways that people react to loss, rejection and exclusion (1994, pp.94–8). Existentially, this is the underground place of grief and shame. Many writers refer to shame – the internalized voice of rejection and the place where people come to believe themselves unworthy to live among their fellow citizens. At the extreme end, Simone Weil speaks of 'affliction', the point at which those in pain and oppression are silenced in their suffering, often not even able to cry out in anger, grief and sorrow (1974, p.182; first published 1962). They seem to know only abandonment.

- Finally, disability is characterized by desire for positive change and striving for emancipation and flourishing. It is seen every day among people living with disability. It is active hope. Since the late 1970s in Australia the majority of people living with disability, some of their families and progressive human services workers have sought a place within (the) community.

Belonging as desire

Community is not simply a place to lay down our heads, but a relational state which brings comfort and support with daily living, friendship, meaningful work, exciting recreation, spiritual renewal, relationships in which we can be ourselves freely with others. And out of this great things may flourish. Perhaps we will begin to feel better about ourselves, to come to know ourselves as honoured, respected, accepted – yes, loved. To be healed from: shame, feeling unworthy, undesirable, ugly, difficult, not smart enough, not sporty enough, not lovely enough. And perhaps we might be freed from our terrible daily fears that it all won't last, that more rejection is written into our lives. Maybe our dreams will no longer be filled with the traumatic fear of others pushing us around.

Perhaps a time will come when we no longer have to protect ourselves from loss and can feel that this place is the place of creation, of recreation, co-creation. Perhaps then our loneliness will fade. Perhaps then we will belong and our gifts (perhaps meagre, perhaps spectacular) freely shared. And from there will flow all the delights and tragedies of a life lived in community, shaped not by exclusion and oppression but by everyday ordinariness (whatever that might be!).

This intersubjective model points us to the importance of relationships – both intimate and remote – as the point at which we both create and alleviate suffering. This is hopeful. It says that all of us can do something that can set free the spirits of those who live with sadness and fear.

Towards spirituality as intersubjective
Promoting isolation or belonging?

I am uncomfortable with a sort of gooey commercialized, universalist notion that 'everyone is spiritual so let's get them doing it'. This assumption is at the heart of tourist brochures offering tantalizing spas and spiritual journeys in the exotic Orient. As one wit recently put it, 'spirituality is the new religion'. To this we could add that spirituality is the new 'simply must have'. Spirituality as a commodity also contributes the therapeutic invasion of spirituality. Commenting on research in spirituality and health, Harry Moody warns: Once the components of positive spirituality are satisfactorily identified, therapists and clinicians will be tempted to 'prescribe' them, even as they now recommend physical and mental medicine and therapy whilst warning against harmful 'snake (sic) medicine' and 'folk cures' (2005, p.33).

One possibly dangerous consequence of seeing spirituality as clinical resource is the lurking concomitant message that those who suffer greatly are spiritually deficient. Many of the people with impairments I know are saying 'don't medicalize our spirits as well as our bodies'. I am not interested in uncritically adding spirituality to the holistic vista of the therapeutically needy.

This leaves me cautious about bringing spirituality into a conversation about disability. But I am not prepared to leave it at that. I am bold enough to claim that understandings of spirituality drawn from the history of religions in dialogue with the work of social movements can be enduring and enriching. Starhawk says:

> Spirituality promotes passivity when the domain of the spirit is defined as outside the world. When this world is the terrain of spirit, we ourselves become actors in the story, and this world becomes the realm in which the sacred must be honored and freedom created. (1987, p.19)

I am interested in developing understandings of spirituality that promote honest engagement; that do not undermine the priority of belonging; that do not sputter out in despair at repeated defeats; that do not climb back onto the armoury of authoritarianism to find some control in the face of intransigent problems; and, finally, that do not turn our attention back to heaven.

I believe that we can incorporate deeply personal aspects of spirituality – its links to transcendence and mystery – with the more social/communal aspects of relationships, the search for peace and justice, as well as aspects of spirituality that speak of global connection. This approach locates sources of strength in our work of embracing socially disparaged people.

In the face of all this evidence, I have come to see that none of these things will overcome threatened belonging until we consciously engage in reconciliation and relationship building. I also believe that looking to resources from the ancient quest for spiritual expression can take us closer to this engagement. The following sections offer significant resources in building an intersubjectively framed liberation spirituality which gives belonging priority.

Encountering the thin places

Many of us, like the poet Adrienne Rich who writes so powerfully of her experience of arthritis, will know of the pain of living with a difficult body. Inga Clendinnen says that falling ill is like falling down Alice's rabbit hole. She opens her account of falling down the rabbit hole, saying

> This is not the story of a medical crisis. If it were, it would be for medicos to write. To lie still as a crusader on a tomb while dreams spin behind closed lids, to surf the tumble of disordered memories as they dolphin away, to feel the mind disintegrate and to fear the disintegration of the self, is to suffer an existential crisis, not a medical one. And to try and understand any of this by transforming inchoate, unstable emotion and sensation into marks on paper is to experience the abyss between fugitive thought, and the words that contain it. (2001, p.1)

The Celts called these rabbit hole experiences 'thin places' in which the manifest world is brought into a close connection with the world of the holy other. Mostly they located these places in woods and streams, but another tradition is emerging which understands thin places as those where great suffering is happening. As physician, Lynette Stevenson says:

> In Celtic mythology, there are pieces of ground considered to be 'thin places' where the measured world comes closest to the infinite. Such places may have been set apart for burial grounds and other ritual sites. The Celtic phrase

describing them derives from the Latin *limen*, a threshold or frontier where two countries meet (the root of 'subliminal'). As physicians, we bear the privilege of escorting patients and families over the thin places. (1998, p.620)

Jeanne Sorrell goes on to say:

In our complex and fast-paced society, we may not take time to explore the thin places where the marginalized dwell... In the midst of the constant noise of our modern world, we fail to create the silence needed for developing practices of intimate listening to the victim's voice. Unless we listen to these voices of diversity, we are likely to remain oblivious to the harm being done in healthcare through unwitting oppression of minorities. (2006, p.152)

Those of us who intervene in the lives of people in suffering, notably here people living with disability – at times of affliction, loss, grief, illness and near death – occupy these thin places and how we handle ourselves there is absolutely important.

Praising paradox

Julian Rappaport (1981) argues that problems within social living are paradoxical because they are made up of real antinomies. Thinking of community living for people of disability, we face real conflicts between seeking empowerment and protection; between our ideals and what is organic; between wanting the moon and having trouble finding an accessible flat. Rappaport says that divergent thought 'is an argument for our work, at both local and social policy level, to recognize and foster the legitimacy of more rather than fewer, different rather than the same ways to deal with problems in living' (p.20).

So we must explore and praise paradox – not to promote a form of paralysis when 'it all seems too big and nothing we do seems to work', but to set us free from seeking once-and-for-all solutions, by taking up Rappaport's challenge to think and act divergently. Here we are not starting with order and seeking to incorporate 'unorder' but starting at unorder and seeking to destabilize all that parades as order.

Enabling engagement

Anthony Kelly depicts our divergent path this way: I am talking about a two-way journey, the trajectory inwards to a fuller sense of self and a deeper spirituality and the circle outwards to a more responsible co-humanity (1989, p.215).

Marjorie Proctor-Smith offers us a dynamic concept of spirituality as 'the string through the middle' that pulls all our disparate parts together. Proctor-Smith arrives at this understanding at the end of a book about women and liturgical traditions. She is critiquing the patriarchal faith traditions. She puts it this way:

> Spirituality, before it is particular disciplines or prayers, is a way of being in the world: a way of living, of knowing, of seeing, of hearing. It is holistic, in the sense that it involves our whole persons: our conscious intellectual life and also our sub-conscious and non-rational life as well; it involves our physical and sensual existence as well as our mental world. Because our spirituality is our way of being in the world, it is also relational and political. It involves the nature of our relationships with others, with God, with the created world and with ourselves. It is thus not individualistic, but corporate; not private but engaged. (1990, p.164)

This dynamic relational view of humanity moves us beyond notions of a fixed essence. It is far from the view that spirit is touched only in our disciplines and rites. It is far from that isolated cosmic mysticism that is so often given prominence in discussions about spirituality. It does not rule out those moments of enlightenment that some are privileged to experience, but it does not say that spirit is touched only in our encounters with the transcendent sacred. Because it is relational and political, it says that our spirit is expanded through the radical revaluing of and encounter with human experience. I agree that it is in the thin places that that encounter is often most richly found with those who are condemned and overlooked. Furthermore, I suggest that this understanding adds depth to the spirituality of those whom we may perceive as the most impaired. Where people cannot speak of matters of the soul, we discover their spirit and are enriched through opening ourselves to intimate encounter with them.

Spirituality seen thus comes with an agenda. It points to a way of being in *this* world, not lifted out of it into another world. It acknowledges that when we are both in and of this world our encounters will include delight and horror, despairs and hopes, elation and suffering. Therefore, it potentially becomes a spirituality of struggle, of confrontation. And it talks not only of resistance but of courage and love.

Embodying 'filoxenia'

As a Greek term, meaning love of the stranger, filoxenia echoes the ancient Hebrew tradition of welcoming the stranger or the sojourner. Filoxenia emerged as a tenet of ancient Greek society because the stranger – however odd they appear to be – might have been one of the gods – not a fellow human either downtrodden or our enemy. However, the contemporary understanding has come to mean hospitality. Walter Brueggemann draws more closely on the Judaic tradition of covenant when he says that

> spirituality is the enterprise of coming to terms with this other in a way that is neither excessively submissive, nor excessively resistant. Such coming to terms is obviously no small matter. For this other is an endless threat to our safety and integrity. This thou always undermines whom we have chosen to be. The presence of the other always reminds us that we are addressed, unsettled, unfinished, underway, not fully whom we intend or pretend to be. (1999, p.2)

Filoxenia is not the easy and pleasant loving of those we are organically drawn to – it is the scary and unsettling love of the person we don't know and won't know unless we move towards them in hospitality or, to use Miroslav Volf's term, embrace. Volf on embrace says that 'the will to give ourselves to others and to "welcome" them, to readjust our identities to make space for them, is prior to any judgment about others, except that of identifying them in their humanity' (1996, p.29).

Identifying with our shared humanity is the first and vital step in the mutual embrace between people with impairments and others. This call is to both sides in the embrace. And it is here that we see most strongly the need to develop a liberation spirituality that speaks for and to people living with disability – a spirituality that offers healing from shame and frees the person to live on in decent, non-humiliating relations.

Risking embrace and drawing strength

These perspectives also show us how, to quote Ali Wurm, to 'love without illusion' (1996, p.49). And all of us who have ever offered or been offered filoxenia know the necessity of doing it without illusion – illusion about our capacity to love and keep on loving; illusion about the impact of our love and work; illusions about the loveliness of the other party. Volf is not advocating that we open ourselves up for further violence, that we should engage in a suicidal throwing ourselves at our killer. Protection is as much a need, in the lives of people living with disability, as empowerment, and we are ethically irresponsible to deny it. Sometimes we might even need to be fierce in our assertion of this protection. Our fears are worthy warnings and wisely attended to. However, they do not have the final say. We also know this from the survivors of abuse, trauma and torture everywhere. We can learn this from people with impairments as they emerge from institutions and seek community. Starhawk reminds us that 'the times may demand courage and self-sacrifice, but we have no spiritual need for martyrdom' (1987, p.22). Yet people living with disability enter our communal living spaces laden with the symbolisms of threat and burden. And if we only see tragedy we will recoil from them as we recoil from the tragedy of decay and death that faces us all.

Where do we gain strength to embrace this other; the courage to risk the powerlessness of reconciliation; the integrity to enter interdependence; the steadiness to endure the pain of the bed of nails? Ultimately the question of drawing strength to do something that might contribute to the end of the cycle of hatred, violence and exclusion that surrounds us will be influenced by culturally determined, personally chosen faith and beliefs. This of course links to the strength that comes from our values, so succinctly put by Starhawk: 'The celebration of life is our value' (1987, p.22).

Liberating spirituality

In response to Adrienne Rich's haunting question 'with whom do you believe your lot is cast?' (1981, p.41) – a question which on the surface contradicts the indiscriminate nature of filoxenia – we can employ Starhawk's 'liberation psychology'. What is true of Starhawk's liberation psychology becomes true of an understanding of spirituality. It becomes an understanding of spirituality that is the 'enemy of sentimentality and of simple solutions' (Winterson 1995). Starhawk says this:

> it must be useful to those who may not have formal education or state approval. Therefore it must be understandable. It is not anti-intellectual, but it realizes that intellect divorced from feeling is part of our pain. Its insights are conveyed in a language that is concrete, a language of poetry, not jargon; of metaphors that clearly are metaphors; a language that refers back to the material world, that is sensual, that speaks of things that we can see and touch and feel. It is a vocabulary not of the elite but of the common, and its concepts can thus be tested by experience. (1987, p.21)

Testing our dreams by experience we also know that community, created through the capacity of thousands to reach beyond themselves and their enclaves to embrace others, has an indefinable, exciting, spontaneous dimension that eludes the scope of even the most dedicated theologians, advocates and community developers. This turn to people generally considered outside the reach of our established concerns is at the heart of filoxenia. Filoxenia offers us embrace with those with whom we might cast our lot: the socially disparaged. I believe, from my own practice and those whom I admire in their vulnerable trusting in the resilience of the human spirit, that this encounter is life-giving for all those who seek it out.

Conclusion: the future

Risking, persisting, celebrating

Sharon Welch reminds us that

> the aims of an ethic of risk may appear modest, yet it offers the potential of sustained resistance against overwhelming odds. The aim is simple – given that we cannot guarantee an end to racism nor the prevention of nuclear war, we can prevent our own capitulation to structural evil. We can participate in a long heritage of resistance, standing with those who have worked for change in the past. We can also take risks trying to create the conditions that will evoke and sustain further resistance. We can help create the conditions necessary for peace and justice, realizing that the choices of others can only be influenced and responded to, never controlled …we cannot make the choices of the next generation; we can only provide a heritage of persistence, imagination and solidarity. (1990, p.22)

This is the final element of liberation spirituality (viewed intersubjectively): the desire to create the conditions for filoxenia to survive into the next generations. We can trust that our intentional involvement to stare down mal-community and to create genuine community, no matter how clumsy and apparently confused, will not guarantee love but it might, just might, contribute to conditions where it can get a toehold. Maybe delight in each other will bring justice and embrace. But until then we work from its second best – a moral sense that all is not right and we must act, urgently, passionately and unstintingly, to build the potential for love to flourish.

Bringing an exploration of an intersubjective, liberation spirituality to building community belonging does not console or soothe. Far from making life easier, it makes it pointier and more disturbing. It does not tell us the way to get living in the world of disability straight. It does not suggest ways to get community relations straight. It does not quieten our worry about whether our intervention is beneficial or harmful. But it is not a narcotic. Those of us with impairments need to own up to the fact that at times we find living achingly difficult and tiring and we need the interventions of others. Our discomfort, our urgency and our not knowing the best solution will keep us vigilant. It will keep us open to those who honestly strive to deal with their reactions. It will respect our exhaustion, it will confront our self-righteousness. It will keep us deeply rooted in a history of solidarity and struggle and keep us from behaving like messiahs. It will give us moments of glory and periods of despondency. It could give us the organically rich lives that we desire for all people...but this may well be the fuel for connection that treats all people as complete human beings. So consciously bringing spirituality to the thin places in search of belonging in community, we strive to know our individual and communal work 'as love made visible' (Walker 1984, p.133).

CHAPTER 9

Scriptural Reminiscence and Narrative Gerontology: Jacob's Wrestling with the Unknown (Genesis 32)

Matthew Anstey

Introduction

Recent research into the phenomenon of ageing has emphasized, among others, two elements, namely, the role of narrative and reminiscence (Haight and Webster 1995; Kenyon, Clark and de Vries 2001) and spiritual care (MacKinlay 2006a). With regard to narrative, although the emphasis tends toward the individual's biography, there is also a recognition of the wider narratives in which the elderly live, such as familial, ethnic, social, and religious. All biographies are embedded in a multiplicity of stories.

MacKinlay's research on elderly spiritual care (2001b, 2002), which also stresses the role of reminiscence, includes as one of many spiritually nurturing activities the reading of sacred texts (e.g. MacKinlay 2006a, pp.36,51,58). However, a review of the literature on ageing and spirituality – and I restrict this study's scope to Christian spirituality – found little specific reflection on the particularities of reading Scripture and ageing (Becker 1986; Bianchi 1992; Clements 1981; Hauerwas *et al.* 2003; Jewell 1999, 2004; Knox 2002; Koenig and Weaver 1998; MacKinlay 2001a; MacKinlay, Ellor and Pickard 2001; Moberg 2001; Morgan 1995).

This is unexpected, due to the important parallels between Scripture as story (both in specific parts and broader framework) and life as story. Reading the Bible is for many elderly people intrinsically bound up with biography at several levels. First, for many their life story includes the whole experience of reading Scripture in various ways: privately, corporately, devotionally, academically. Their memory of these countless acts of reading is a source of meaning. Second, for many the core narratives, such as Exodus, creation, Christmas, Easter, the Burning Bush, the sacrifice of Isaac, have an authority (however defined) much greater than other non-biographical narratives, such as those found in literature, theatre, cinema, popular culture, or elsewhere. For instance, MacKinlay (2001a, p.89) cites a survey in the USA in which '38 percent of people at senior centres reported reading the Bible or other religious material on a daily basis'. This indicates the centrality of sacred story to the religious life of the elderly.

Third, and most importantly, for many the scriptural story is their story. Rost (2005, p.129) writes 'The Scriptures tell me that my story is part of a much longer, historical, eschatological, universal Story. I am part of a people who are all on the same pilgrimage toward communion with God and, in God, with each other.'

There have been a few publications exploring this connection. Jamieson (2005) provides a short non-academic guide to spiritual reminiscence. This guide is valuable for small groups in a parish or community setting in facilitating the exploration of life stories and their meaning in light of Scripture.

Achenbaum and Modell (1999) draw interesting parallels between the life journeys of Abraham and Sarah (Genesis 12–25) and the contemporary thinkers Erik and Joan Erikson. This article illustrates that sacred and contemporary stories can illuminate one another, but offers no methodology for such and concentrates on the biographical side.

Eisenhandler (1999) presents a case study in which twelve women read weekly in a group three books and an anthology for twelve weeks. Most of the readings were non-religious, but provided an impetus for discussions of matters transcendent. Eisenhandler notes the dynamics of *reading* together and of reading *reflectively*. I will return to Eisenhandler's insights in the final section of this chapter. Koenig unfortunately groups prayer and Bible-reading together as 'religious activity', and thus overlooks the distinctive features of Scripture-reading (1994, pp.258–261, 452–456).

Rost (2005) discusses the relationship of sacred to autobiography, drawing heavily from Gerkin (1984). He asserts the significance of the Scriptures in Judeo-Christian spirituality, as a story of God's dealings with His people that definitively shapes their life together (pp.124–5). Thus God's people are constantly engaged in *remembering*, not only autobiography, but remembering their participation in God's story, with all its attendant promises, dramas, ambiguities, and so forth (p.125). Furthermore, biography for many includes 'sacred remembrance, i.e., the searching of one's memories for the presence and purpose of God' (p.126). Rost notes that sacred stories and life stories illuminate each other:

> The Scriptures become both a role model and a motivator for us to remember, share and interpret our own and each other's stories. And, conversely, the more we are in touch with our own stories and their meanings, the more alive and powerful the stories, images and metaphors of the Scriptures become. (p.127)

Rost discerns, in different language, the intrinsic connection between sacred and personal narrative: 'the process of reminiscence is impoverished by the absence of the Scriptures' (p.129). Thus for Rost, interpretation of auto-biography goes hand-in-hand with interpretation of Scripture, co-contributing to the hermeneutical task of pastoral care for the elderly. This does not exclude other narrative resources, but recognizes that for those elderly who identify themselves as belonging to religious communities the sacred texts are qualitatively distinct contributors in the formation of self-as-narrative.

Thus scriptural stories are not simply 'adjuncts to reminiscence theory' (Burnside 1995, p.153). They do not simply offer a means of arriving at narrative truth by indirection (sometimes called 'a third thing', e.g. Palmer 2004 in spiritual direction); rather, they are intrinsic to autobiography itself, providing crucial (sub-)plots to issues of faith, morality, purpose, the after-life, belonging, beauty, reconciliation, and so forth.

More broadly, the significance of narrative to self-identity has been approached from many angles, such as philosophical (Ricoeur 2004), theological (Goldberg 1991; Hauerwas and Jones 1989) and psychiatric (Meares 2000, 2005), and journals such as the *International Journal of Narrative Therapy and Community Work* are devoted to therapeutic dimensions of story.

Thus narrative broadly construed appears as a major conceptual category in a large number of disciplines. This study makes a case for and a case study of the specific link between scriptural narrative and narrative gerontology.

The possibility of scriptural reminiscence: a case study based on Genesis 32

I want to proceed now in the argument through a case study of interpretation, by examining the ways a pivotal story from the Old Testament potentially sheds light on and contributes to elderly biography. I do so as an expert not in ageing but in Hebrew narrative, which requires the same level of care and sophistication in interpretation as does a person's life.

However, with my readership in mind, I will re-present the story in a non-technical style, much the same way it could be used as a spiritual reading in a senior's setting. I will suggest in the final section that *scriptural reminiscence* could be used to delineate the unique place that Scripture plays in reminiscence for elderly persons for whom Scripture is intrinsic to their biography.

Scholarly works I consulted in my interpretation of this text include Brodie (2001), Kass (2003), Kugel (2003), Sarna (1989), Wenham (1994), and Westermann (1985). There is disagreement over where this story starts, and my choice of Genesis 32:22 (32:21 in English) as a starting point is less commonly held.

Preamble

The figure of the patriarch Jacob, one of Scripture's most intricately sketched characters, looms large in the second half of Genesis. From his unusual birth to his controversial final words before death, Jacob's life has fascinated readers, in no small part due to the story's brutal honesty, brimming as it is with deception, grief, trauma, and estrangement.

The reader, however, has a demanding task in ascertaining how the multifarious chapters of Jacob's life inform Judeo-Christian spirituality, let alone spirituality pertaining to ageing and disability, for, as in most Hebrew Bible narratives, aphorisms and/or happy endings are rarely found. Thus the reader, like Jacob, must learn to wrestle with the text patiently and attentively to discern its deeper significances.

The story of Jacob's wrestling provides a vignette of Jacob's entire life, a life dominated by the pursuit of what I call the *elusive blessing*, which comes to Jacob unexpectedly after a dark night of leaving, limping, and letting go.

Leaving, limping, and letting go: Jacob's wrestle for the elusive blessing

Scene 1 – Genesis 32:22–25a [Eng. 21–24a]

So the gift crossed over before Jacob's face; and he himself spent that night in the camp. And he arose in the night and took his two wives, his two slavegirls, and his eleven children, and crossed over the ford of the Jabbok. He took them and he made them cross over the stream, and he made everything that he had cross over. And Jacob was left alone.

Like many a good story, the beginning is crucial and here is no exception. Five words set the scene – gift, crossing over, face, night, alone.

Word one: gift. The gift sets the context: Jacob has sent ahead a gift, more like a bribe, to his estranged brother Esau, whom he has not seen in decades. The storyteller is thus setting the story against the background of relationship discord. It is brimming with the anxiety of a hoped-for reconciliation, a fearful longing. 'Will Esau accept me?', Jacob wonders.

Word two: crossing over. This is mentioned four times in scene 1. Here we are at a river, a boundary marker, and first the gift crosses over. We know from verses 15–16 that this gift includes 550 animals: goats, sheep, camels, cows, and donkeys. Now that's a gift, and indicates just how worried Jacob is about pleasing Esau. Secondly his family crosses over. This is repeated, 'he made them cross over.' And finally, everything he has crosses over.

Jacob is stripped down to the bare essentials. In the shadowy night to follow, nothing, not even his family, can accompany him. The crossing over symbolizes a removal of all that Jacob has acquired in life through hard work, but also trickery and deception – remember, his name, Jacob, means 'deceiver' (Genesis 25:26). Jacob parts with all that he has used to build his identity and to secure his place in the world, all of which won't matter in the coming tempest.

Word three: face. The gift crossed over before Jacob's *face*. He watched it go past as the sun was setting, before the blustery stranger arrived in the night. Was there a tightness of anxious worry in his brow? Or perhaps a shoulder-sagging resignation, as he realized the futility of all this stuff? And with all his material possessions gone, what new face might appear in the now-vacant space?

Word four: night. At this point, the lights go out. Night is the time of poor vision, the time of elevated fear, the time of compromised ability. Night is ripe with danger. And this night, we are to surmise, Jacob couldn't sleep. He got up during the night, and sent all his worldly possessions across the river. It is as if he could not bear to be with anyone in his moment of suspenseful waiting. Jacob, like all of us, knows when he needs what my young daughter Tayah calls PS – *personal space.* 'Just leave me be!', Jacob pleads before a starry sky.

Word five: alone. 'And Jacob was left alone.' This word was last used of Adam, when God declared it was not good for Adam to be alone (Genesis 2:18). It is not wholesome, satisfying, nor complete, for a person to be alone (in the sense of having no relationships).

Jacob chose the isolation into which God appeared, but to some it comes unbeckoned – addictions, accidents, atrocious mistakes, and of course ageing – they can all leave us so lonely we feel like we will seep away unnoticed like liquid into the ground.

Five words:

Gift – Jacob has given one. Will he receive one?

Crossing over – Everything except Jacob has crossed over. Will Jacob also cross over?

Face – Nothing now stands before Jacob's face. Will someone appear?

Night – His moment of greatest vulnerability. Will someone take advantage of him?

Alone – Our greatest fear. Who am I when the lights are out and all have left me?

Scene 2 – Genesis 32:25b–30 [Eng. 24b–29]
Scene 2a – 25b–26 [Eng. 24b–25]

And a man wrestled with him until daybreak. And the man saw that he did not prevail against him, and he struck him on the hip socket; and Jacob's hip was put out of joint as he wrestled with him.

Unannounced, a protagonist appears on the scene whose identity is uncertain, but who at the very last moment turns out to be God. Isn't this how many of us experience the divine – our suspicions are raised, we grope for clues; we ask, 'Is that you God?' And then, at the moment of recognition, God frustratingly slips away again.

This God-stranger wrestles with Jacob through the evening. Jacob did not decline this nocturnal struggle. They were, we realize, evenly matched. God is presented neither as a bully nor a doormat. God meets Jacob on his shadowy night at the level of his capacity to resist.

Yet here the mystery deepens, as the stranger cannot overcome Jacob, so he injures him, dislocating his hip in some way.

What will happen now in this dangerous fusion of wrestling skin-on-skin?

Scene 2b – 27–30 [Eng. 26–29]

And he said, 'Let me go, for the day is breaking.' And Jacob said, 'I will not let you go, unless you bless me.' And he said to him, 'What is your name?' And he said, 'Jacob.' And the man said, 'You shall no longer be called Jacob, but Israel, for you have wrestled with God and with humans, and have prevailed.' And Jacob asked him, 'Please tell me your name.' And he said, 'Why is it that you ask my name?' And he blessed him there.

Such a short conversation, yet, to put it mildly, such an astonishing conversation, rarely bettered in all of sacred Scripture.

> We, like the hero Jacob are in the dark about the identity of his opponent, the reason for his attack, the nature of the wound, the significance of the outcome, the meaning of Jacob's new name, and the importance of the story for the rest of Jacob's life – and for his people Israel. At no point in the entire Jacob saga are we in more need of careful interpretation and searching reflection. (Kass 2003, p.456)

And the stranger said, 'Let me go! For the day is breaking!' Jacob, who has let go of everything, has found something worth holding onto. Jacob has found himself in the fight of his life and he's not going to let this one get away.

So he screams at his opponent in their entanglement: *'I won't let you go until you bless me!'*

All of Jacob's life can be compressed into this one word: blessing.

He stole a blessing, as you may remember, from his brother (Genesis 27), but it was not his own idea, it was his mother's. But he went ahead and stole it anyway; in the 'darkness' of his father's blindness he received his first blessing. But for this blessing, the blessing Jacob *wants*, darkness is still the context.

Jacob realizes that this stranger is not an ordinary man – he is God and rule number one is, if you get God in a headlock, don't let go! – what an opportunity of a lifetime! 'I won't let you go until you bless me!' '*I've* figured out who you are and *I've* got the upper hand', Jacob thinks to himself. 'You said so yourself when you revealed your weakness, saying "Let me go!". That'll teach you, Mr God-posing-as-stranger, not to make yourself vulnerable.'

And so the God-man said something disarmingly simple, 'What is your name?' 'What is your name? Tell me who you are. You want a blessing, Jacob, then you're going to have to tell me your name first. I don't want your share portfolio, your blood-type, your Myers-Briggs results, your Functional Autonomy Measurement Score. I don't want to know about the money you've gained, the prizes you've won, the degrees you've earned, the mountains you've climbed. What I do want is this: tell me who you are? I want to know you better.'

This is where we must read very carefully – this question must have set off a depth charge in Jacob, because Jacob has heard this question before!

Many years ago, as a young man at his dying father's side, dressed up as his brother to deceive, his father asked him, *'Who are you, my son?'* (Genesis 27:18) and Jacob – whose name means *deceiver* – deceitfully answered 'Esau!'

And so now, when asked 'What is your name?', Jacob answers honestly, 'I am Jacob. I am a deceiver.'

To receive the blessing he longs for, Jacob must admit finally who he is. Jacob must finally whisper his true name.

And then the elusive blessing comes: 'Your name shall be Israel, for you have struggled with God and people and have prevailed.'

The conversation continues. Jacob, God bless him (!), wants more; Jacob wants to upsize this spiritual meal-deal. 'Please tell me your name!' Jacob wants to capture the moment forever by getting a handle on the divine, 'Please tell me your name!' He wants some secret knowledge about God, some name that, like a genie in a bottle, will force God to appear whenever Jacob wants. But the God-stranger replies, 'Why do you ask for my name?' – which is polite God-talk for 'Sorry, Jacob, but no cigar!' And so God blessed him there. Jacob didn't receive any *thing*, but he did receive a new name and a limp, a disability no less.

The limp is a new way of being in the world, a new way of being recognized, of journeying, a reminder of his brokenness. Jacob's lonely struggle that one long evening is converted into a lifelong struggle in his walking.

Scene 3 – Genesis 32:31–33 [Eng. 30–32]

So Jacob called the place Peniel (The-Face-of-God), saying, 'For I have seen God face to face, and yet my life is preserved.' The sun rose upon him as he crossed over Peniel [Hebrew: Penuel, a variant of Peniel], limping because of his hip. Therefore to this day the Israelites do not eat the thigh muscle that is on the hip socket, because he struck Jacob on the hip socket at the thigh muscle.

Our crafty storyteller brings together in the conclusion the five words we met in the introduction – gift, face, crossing over, night, alone – and each is transformed.

- Jacob's strings-attached *gift*, replaced by God's free gift of blessing.

- Jacob's *face* in front of which all his life passed, replaced by God's face, up close and personal.

- Jacob's lack of *crossing over*, replaced by his crossing over to the waiting community.

- Jacob's *night*, replaced by the new day.

- Jacob's *aloneness*, replaced by a divine enveloping.

To this list, five more transformations can be added:

- Jacob's *name*, Deceiver, replaced by Israel, which means God-Wrestler.

- Jacob's *place*, Jabbok, replaced by Peniel, God's presence.

- Jacob's brisk *stride*, replaced by a cautious limp.

- Jacob's relentless *grip* on the stranger, replaced by a letting-go of the unknowable.

- Jacob's life-sapping worldly *possessions*, displaced by life-giving blessing.

Moreover, the narrator not only repeats here the word cross over, for the fifth and final time: 'Jacob crossed over Peniel limping', he also adds another allusion: Jacob, on whom God inflicts a limp *tsala'* (in Hebrew), to make him whole in *solitude*, is like Adam, from whom God took a rib *tsela'* (Genesis 2:21–22) to make him whole in relationship. Rib *tsela'*, limp *tsala'* – we are made whole when God touches us.

It is as though the transformative forces released in Jacob's life flow into his surroundings – he gains a new name, a new way of being, and a new place. We have been warned: when we enter the brawling darkness of an unyielding grappling with God, anything and everything might change.

And then, the story ends in typical Old Testament style, with a reference to an aspect of daily life: 'Don't eat the thigh muscle!' The almost mythical story of Jacob's wrestling is anchored in the mundane, the daily life of eating and childbirth, olive trees and threshing floors. This narrative movement mimics our lives, replete with the ordinary, yet dappled with unexpected flecks of divine. Eating with friends and wrestling with angels – we separate them narratalogically at our own risk.

Interpretive possibilities

I have retold this story carefully, imaginatively and evocatively to demonstrate its profound interpretive potential. Because the story deals with ultimate questions, some may say philosophical and/or religious questions, it can play a particularly insightful role in spiritual reminiscence.

As I mentioned above, scriptural reminiscence might be appropriate for the combination of this kind of reading coupled with reflective practice, defined as *reminiscence that involves the reading and interpreting of biography in the light of Scripture, in recognition of its unique place in the self-as-narrative of religious elderly.*

Let me illustrate this by considering briefly three aspects of Genesis 32. Again, I do not claim any expertise in the area of narrative and therapy or self-identity, so my suggestions derive from my reading of the Hebrew story (and my participation in Christian communities as an ordained Anglican) rather than from clinical practice.

The possibility of scriptural reminiscence

Blessing

This story, indeed, the whole life of Jacob is tied up with blessing, a rich and nuanced word in Christian thinking. In popular culture, blessing is strongly associated with material and/or medical wellness (e.g. Dictionary.com Unabridged n.d.). Thus blessing as an interpretative lens for the elderly is very pertinent, because in ageing wellness is often in decline and acquisition of material possessions is less significant.

Blessings are often presented in Christian congregations as being fairly immediate, accessible, attainable. Blessings are things we can aspire to; even politicians promise to give us blessings these days, let alone priests and doctors and nurses. Such easily gained blessing, we are led to believe, comes when we get things – blessing is all about *stuff*, stuff God and faith (and hard work) gives us.

But in Jacob's wrestling, a story that exposes the meaning of blessing, all of Jacob's stuff is on the other side of the river! The blessing comes at the climax of the story when Jacob admits his true name (representing his true self). Thus to bless someone in this story is to name someone, to reveal their true nature, who they are and who they are to become.

Hence I subtitled this chapter 'Jacob's wrestling with the unknown' precisely because it presents a counter-narrative to the popular – even in Christian churches – narrative of easy blessing.

Transformation

I listed in scene 3 the ten things that change in this story: gift, face, crossing over, night, aloneness, name, place, stride, grip, and possessions. The narrator leaves virtually nothing unchanged by this exhausting encounter with the divine. As is well documented, ageing is characterized by great change. It can come in one evening, as for Jacob, or it can be gradual. The beauty of story is that the narrative time, however compressed, can be mapped onto an endless variety (and number) of biographical times. A careful reading of Jacob's story by and with elderly people could investigate the way this story illuminates the experience of 'everything's changing' for the elderly.

Letting go and not-knowing

In the centre of the story, verse 30, Jacob asks a question: 'Please tell me your name.'

But God never answers the question, instead replying with another question, 'Why do you ask my name?' Jacob is then blessed and the God-stranger leaves. But we also know that the stranger couldn't overcome Jacob, so the careful reader will infer that *Jacob must have let go*. What we have here, in the centre of Jacob's struggle with God, is an unanswered question, followed by a letting-go of God and so a letting-go of the need for an answer. We could express this as follows: *at the heart of every person's life of faith is an unanswered question.*

In a senior's context, it is easy to think of unanswered questions: Why do I have to suffer this terrible disability? Why did those who were supposed to love and nurture me fail to do so? Why did someone I love so dearly have to die? Why has my deepest desire in the world not been granted?

Again, the astute reader will notice that the blessing comes *after* the letting-go (scene 2b). Hence we can tie these threads together: blessing is elusive precisely because paradoxically it comes when we let go, accepting that its secret answer will not be surrendered.

There are other aspects of this evocative story that could provide angles on self-as-narrative, such as the motif of darkness, of limping and slowing down, of uncertainty in the identity of the stranger-God, of the movement from community to solitude and back to community.

Conclusions

I have suggested two things in this chapter:

1. That spiritual reminiscence cannot simply include 'Bible-reading' as a spiritual 'activity', on a par with church attendance, liturgy, and so forth. It is qualitatively different, with respect to its embeddedness *as* sacred story *in* life story. I suggest a distinct place for scriptural reminiscence, the reading and interpreting of biography in the light of Scripture, in recognition of its unique place in the self-as-narrative of religious elderly.

2. That when the interpretation of Scripture is treated with the same level of sophistication as is practised with the 'ageing' disciplines, such as narrative gerontology, a greater benefit is gained, due to the subtleties and ambiguities and questions revealed in the text, which opens up more interpretative possibilities for the readers.

Hence narrative gerontology with religious elderly faces two tasks: first, as a *retrospective* life-mapping task, it needs to find ways of measuring degree of significance of non-autobiographical narratives such as sacred texts, and to supplement quantity of 'religious activity' with quality of significant non-biographical text interpretation. Second, as a *prospective* form of care-giving, carers should be seeking actively to assist the deep, reflective (individual and corporate) reading of sacred stories, trusting the stories' potential to facilitate the (re-)formation of meaning, which can lead to re-storying, what Gerkin calls 'changing the story' (1984, pp.143–76), in a way that maintains respectfully autobiographical integrity but allows alternative, imaginative understandings of life events and beliefs in the journey toward personal wholeness.

Scriptural reminiscence, if as a practice it gains currency, thus requires the nurturing of practices of reflective reading. Eisenhandler (1999, p.3) correctly notes the pre-modern practice of such, developed in monastic settings and often called *lectio divina* (divine reading) or *ruminatio* (rumination). Scriptural reminiscence offers an interesting possibility for further research from theoretical, methodological and pastoral perspectives.

In Gerkin's 'hermeneutics of selfhood' (1984, p.102), this dialectical contribution of scriptural narratives to self-narratives is subsumed under the broader category of 'interpretations of faith and culture'. He is worth quoting at length in conclusion (pp.103–4, emphasis mine):

> From this direction come most particularly those mythic and symbolic interpretative patterns by which a tradition or way of life is shaped over time in a given locale ... They not only provide languages by which behaviours and relationships are given meaning, but also exert a powerful force in shaping the individuals' perceptions of self and world. They tell us what thoughts and behaviours should be assigned guilty, accusatory meaning and what should receive commendation. They define for us what relationships should be and why. *In large part the individual's sense of self and world are bestowed by the interpretations of faith traditions and culture.*

Note

Dr Matthew P. Anstey is the recipient of an Australian Research Council Postdoctural Fellowship (2006–2009, project number DP0663901).

CHAPTER 10

Tracing Rainbows through the Rain: Addressing the Challenge of Dementia in Later Life

Malcolm Goldsmith

George Matheson (1842–1906), a Church of Scotland minister, wrote the hymn 'O Love that wilt not let me go' after he became blind. He wrote it on the eve of his sister's wedding as he remembered with pain how his own fiancée had broken off their engagement when she had learned of his impending blindness. He said that he wrote the hymn in a matter of minutes, as though the words came to him from beyond himself. It is a hymn that many people love as they struggle to hold on to the mystery of life when their experiences seem to deny all that is good and wholesome. In this chapter I will use a few lines of that hymn as a sort of refrain, coming back to them from time to time.

> I trace the rainbow through the rain
> And feel the promise is not vain
> That morn shall tearless be.

The rainbow is a biblical image of hope and over the centuries many people have found comfort and hope in its symbolic meaning. In the story of the flood, the rain symbolizes all those forces which can destroy us, our sense of worth and dignity and above all our sense of hope. The story of the flood represents, in symbolic terms, the titanic struggle between good and evil, between life and death, between hope and despair. In other stories rain can symbolize life and health and renewal but in this story it symbolizes that which would destroy us and the rainbow comes with its message of hope.

There are, of course, many other images that have been used over the years to portray the experience or reality of hope. The new dawn, dispelling the darkness of the night; the beauty of the butterfly emerging from the dark imprisonment of the chrysalis; the young chicken pecking its way through the egg shell and experiencing the light and space of its new world; the shoots which spring up from the ground after the seed has lain hidden beneath the surface of the soil through all the long winter months.

There are stories of people and events which can also convey a sense of hope. The composer Händel was in deep personal and financial trouble but from within the situation he was able to write the music to the Hallelujah chorus. Martin Luther King on one occasion wrote about the experience of being imprisoned 'if he puts you in jail you transform that jail from a dungeon of shame to a haven of human freedom and dignity'. Each day, as we read the newspapers we come across stories of amazing acts of love or generosity which stand out like beacons in the midst of all the stories of destruction and despair. In 2003 a Jewish student from Britain on a visit to Tel Aviv was killed by a Palestinian suicide bomber. His family donated an organ from his body to save the life of a Palestinian girl. More recently, the family of a Palestinian boy shot by an Israeli soldier donated his organs to a number of people including two Israeli children; without that gift they would have surely died. Picasso's majestic picture painted after the bombing of Guernica is a huge painting showing death and destruction, everything tumbling apart, disjointed and, at first glance, impossible to make any sense of. But there, within this great representation of pain and grief and barbarity, it is possible to see a tiny, fragile symbol of hope, as a small shoot bearing a leaf of new life grows out of the wooden handle of a broken sword.

> I trace the rainbow through the rain
> And feel the promise is not vain
> That morn shall tearless be.

All these examples touch our deepest emotions and very often we are unable to find ways of expressing what we experience. At times like these, very often music, poetry or art are essential means of communication. A touch, a smile or a tear may be more understandable than a thousand words. Just how we experience and reflect upon these deepest emotions, how we seek to make sense of the world and how we endeavour to communicate to others how we feel and what we hope and strive for, is the raw material for what we loosely call 'spirituality'. It is our attempt to make some sort of sense of the mystery of life, with its beauty and joys but also with its pain and suffering. People with different sorts of personality will often experience these things in different ways; some people may espouse religious language to describe or reflect on them whilst others will not find that sort of language helpful or appropriate.

Whatever language is used, there seems to be a universal desire to make sense of our situation and to find signs of hope when our surroundings threaten to diminish or destroy us. Some would say that such a longing was archetypal and that it was nature's way of helping us to survive; others would point to God's promise that in the end all will be made good. It is possible to yearn for, to believe in, a future without tears, without necessarily believing in God or being a religious person; such feelings are universal. Similarly, the morn can hold the promise of hope without us necessarily believing that it is a promise from God, although many people would want to understand it in that way. As we struggle with the mystery of life and death, a great many people have found comfort in the words of the hymn and the symbol of the rainbow.

In this chapter I want to reflect upon the experience of dementia, both for the person with dementia and also for those who care for people with dementia, and explore whether it is possible to find any seeds of hope within this devastating illness.

Many people will find that this description rings true to their own experience:

> The person you loved has gone. There is no-one left to talk to, there is no companionship any more, but at the same time there is a highly demanding person who needs to be fed and dressed and cleaned up. This same loved-one has become (in some cases) unreasonable and cantankerous and unable even to say thank you. At times he doesn't recognize members of his own family and orders them about as if they were servants. His wife is a stranger, whilst there are moments when he mistakes his daughter for his wife.

> For some carers there comes the point where they feel that they have been bereaved. The body may require attention, but the real person has departed. Now there may be a permanent feeling of bereavement; the tears may flow, but the period of grieving may be long and drawn out. The funeral service may be many months or years away and when death eventually comes, there may be no more tears to shed. (Sutcliffe 1988 p.43)

Despite all the advances that are being made in understanding the causes and pathways of dementia and despite the real progress that is being made in learning more about what it means to have dementia or to care for someone with dementia, it is still a terrible illness. It is terminal; we know of no cure; it is progressive, it gets steadily worse and it can last for many years. It is a frightening journey that the person with dementia is taking and it can be devastatingly difficult and tiring for those who walk alongside them.

Henry Scott-Holland (1910) was a Canon at St Paul's Cathedral in London before becoming Regius Professor of Divinity at Oxford. Whilst in London he preached a sermon about death 'The King of Terrors' which contained words often quoted at funerals even today, but they are words which I have always found quite problematic. 'Death is nothing at all, I have only slipped away into the next room'. I have never been able to accept that view. I can understand that its purpose is to try and minimize the grief of the mourners, but to me death is something that is very real, very tangible and invariably painful and sad. For the person who dies, it is the end of their life, and for those who mourn, it represents a huge change. I know that sometimes death, when it comes, comes as a welcome release, but to say that it is nothing at all denies the reality of death and the authenticity of my grief. Similarly with dementia, we have to face up to the reality of the seriousness of the diagnosis and the awfulness of many of the consequences, but need this be the final word about dementia? Is it possible, whilst accepting the general truth of the description I have just quoted, to stop and draw a caveat – to say that this may be true but it is not the whole truth? Is it possible to find hope within such a situation of despair? Is it possible to 'trace the rainbow through the rain and feel the promise is not vain that morn shall tearless be'?

I have sometimes heard people speak about a 'wilderness experience' when talking about dementia. It is an apt image, for the wilderness brings to mind an inhospitable terrain, a sense of being lost and the constant fear of running out of resources. There is the scorching sun by day and the marked contrast of the cold dark night which can remind us of the contrasts and the fluctuations we sometimes know and experience in dementia care – sometimes knowing and at other times not knowing, sometimes here and at other times absent. The wilderness, the desert, has so often been a place of abandonment and there is little wonder that it has so often appeared as an image within the Bible. It is a place of testing, which is one reason why the image so often resonates with people involved in dementia care. Joyce Huggett writes of the desert in this way (1988, p.117):

> [it] is a place of stripping and a place of terror, a place of wonder and a place of promise, a place of testing and a place of paralysis of the soul. The desert may be a situation of hopelessness, a state of mental anguish, deep down loneliness or emotional emptiness. The desert, alternatively, can be a place where God whispers words of tenderness, a place where we meet with our creator in a life-changing way.

The writer of the book Deuteronomy must have had this in mind when he wrote

> In a desert land he found him,
> in a barren and howling waste.

> He shielded him and cared for him;
> he guarded him as the apple of his eye. (32:10)

And so we are confronted by this paradox again, being lost and being found, being desolate and being cared for, like the rainbow in the rain.

There is also another way of looking at dementia and it is this other way that I now want to focus upon. By way of introduction let me quote from a novel:

> It was now four years since the dementia was diagnosed. It seemed both as yesterday and also as though it had always been the case. There is no space for time in dementia, time stands still. Time is a commodity for those who are busy, who live by diaries, calendars and clocks. You need none of these when you just exist, when your days pass almost unnoticed, each one there to be lived through, full of incidents, full of pauses. Time becomes irrelevant, what is it but the passing of days, the journeys of the earth around the sun, the changing of the seasons. Time is not life. Life is something entirely different. Bill knew that, so did Victoria. Life was about the smiles they exchanged without the need for words. Life was about the way Bill massaged her hands with cream, brushed her hair, cleaned her teeth and ensured that day by day she continued to look good and wore clothes which suited her. Life was about having a grandchild on your knee even though you did not understand the relationship or remember the name. Life was being surrounded by people who loved you and whose love was unconditional. (Goldsmith 2007)

'There is no space for time in dementia, time stands still.' Or perhaps there are different times, different phases that people with dementia and their carers pass through, each possessing the possibilities for growth and nourishment whilst also containing the seeds of possible despair and dissolution. Below I describe a series of experiences which are common as people address the challenge of dementia in later life, although they do not necessarily occur in the order in which I am setting them down. In each instance I am exploring whether there are any symbols, stories, metaphors or myths which can help us to understand the situation better and whether there are any grounds for hope.

Whenever we enter into another person's experiences of suffering, we need to tread very carefully for we tread upon sacred ground. When we begin to open up the experience of pain and suffering, sadness and despair, we are entering into spaces of great tenderness and privacy. It is with this approach that I want to explore some of the experiences that people with dementia and their carers have shared with me. I am conscious of a great invisible fellowship of those who suffer and grieve. They are not alone, isolated individuals, they are part of a great company whose tears and laughter, pain and strength enable them to cope against almost unbelievable odds.

The experience of dementia as a time of waiting

So often I am asked 'how long?', but there are no easy answers to such a question. It is a time of waiting. There are things in life that we cannot rush, they must take their natural course; whether it be a pregnancy or a seed in the ground, there is a time and a season. As a child I remember wanting to hurry Christmas along, or my birthday – no doubt entirely centred upon my expectation of gifts, but no matter how strong my longing, the time was not affected by what I felt or thought. Time has its own momentum. A few years ago I knew that I had to undergo heart surgery and I had to wait – and wait. A date had to be set for the operation and I could neither reduce nor extend that time; I had to let it take its course.

Often it is not the waiting itself which is so difficult as much as the sense of not knowing. How long will the waiting be? There is a story in the Old Testament, in the Hebrew Scriptures, about the prophet Elijah having to endure a drought. He went out into the wilderness to await a word from the Lord. We are told that he waited for a very long time and it was three years before he received any sign from God. Three years alone, and in the wilderness, in a time of drought. How did he cope? How do we cope?

We need to develop a new attitude towards time, stressing not the length of days but the quality of life. But even that is not easy when it is the quality of life which is itself being threatened, day after day after day. I remember hearing a radio programme several years ago in which the former England cricketer Geoffrey Boycott talked about how cricketers' minds worked when they were amassing a large score. He said it was necessary to break it down into small units. They batted until the next significant number of runs was reached – 10, 25 or 50 – or they looked towards staying at the crease until lunchtime or the tea interval. 'Don't think in terms of hundreds,' he said, 'think in terms of tens or in terms of fifteen-minute spells.' Similarly, with dementia care it is a question of looking towards the next little milestone, today or tomorrow, this afternoon or this evening. The long walk always begins and continues with a small step. In this way it might be easier for us to seize the moments of meaning, of recognition or laughter. In this way we might begin to experience what has been called 'the sacrament of the present moment'. We live for today. Not regretting yesterday nor anticipating tomorrow, as I read somewhere – yesterday is history, tomorrow is mystery and today is a gift, which is why it is called the present.

The experience of dementia as a time of disempowerment

It can be a time of great frustration, anger and resentment. Not being able to do what was previously possible is a real challenge. How can people focus upon what is still possible rather than dwell upon what is no longer possible? Do we rage on, as in Dylan Thomas's poem about his father's death (Thomas 1971), or find ways of accepting gracefully what can no longer be done? On the other hand, can we accept that it is perfectly acceptable to rage just as it is acceptable to remain calm, even though our raging may be much more difficult for other people to cope with? Who would not rage or want to rage at times?

Again, using a story from the Bible, the time when the Hebrew people were perhaps most disempowered was when they were defeated in battle by the might of Babylon, Jerusalem was in ruins and the Temple destroyed. People were marched off, hundreds of miles, into exile in a strange land. It was a land foreign to them in every respect and, crucially, it was a land outside the power and influence, so they thought, of their God. 'By the waters of Babylon we sat down and wept… How shall we sing the Lord's song in a strange land?' (Psalm 137:1, 4). But it was there, in the poverty and impotence of their exile, that they wrote some of the most beautiful of all the writings in the Hebrew Scriptures (including the famous Suffering Servant songs) and it was there, hundreds of miles away from their destroyed Temple, that they discovered a new understanding about the nature of God and their own destiny.

It is possible for something new to break through even in times of the utmost disempowerment. For those who are carers this is most important, for sometimes we allow ourselves to become disempowered. We can disempower ourselves by thinking that there is nothing we can do, but that is rarely the case. Beethoven wrote some of his finest music when he was totally deaf; Martin Luther King turned his prison cell from a dungeon of despair into a haven of righteousness; and the Scottish minister wrote, from his condition of blindness and a broken heart,

> I trace the rainbow through the rain
> And feel the promise is not vain
> That morn shall tearless be.

There is enough disempowerment in the experience of dementia without us adding to it, but to be positive and creative in such a situation is incredibly difficult. We can take heart from the many people who are able to do it, not because they are strong or heroic but because they are human and they reveal something of the innate wonder of what it is to be human.

There is something about humanity which defies so much of what would diminish it. I am reminded of the little poem:

> Sometimes I picture myself
> like a candle.
> I used to be a candle about eight feet tall –
> burning bright.
> Now, every day I lose
> a little bit of me.
> Someday the candle will be
> very small.
> But the flame will be
> just as bright. (Noon 2003, reproduced with kind permission.)

The experience of dementia as a time of disengagement, isolation and tiredness

It is said that a person with dementia often seems to drift away for a while, being there but at the same time not being there. They lose interest in the world around them. These times can vary in length but they are times of disengagement, as though the person is on a journey into a strange land in which the carer cannot accompany them. It is an exaggeration of a tendency that we all have experienced as we move on from one stage of life to another; a process in which we disengage from the concerns of one stage, as we engage with the concerns of the next. There is invariably a sense of loss in these transitions but we cannot hang on to what was, we have to be open to what is emerging. It can be a difficult and painful time. It can leave the person with dementia and their carers feeling very isolated, from each other and from other people. One carer described it in this way:

> when you feel that not only does no-one understand but you get the feeling (rightly or wrongly) that friends and relations and even one's own church do not want to understand or even know about what you are both experiencing – it makes for a very rough and weary road to follow. You have no previous experience to fall back on and no light at the end of the tunnel. (Jeremiah 2003, p.25)

'A rough and weary road': weariness is one of the most often quoted feelings of those who care. Many people battle against sheer exhaustion, with night after night of broken sleep. They often feel that their plight is not understood and they are probably right, for who can fully understand the burdens and fears and weariness of another? Carers often speak of an overwhelming tiredness and yet they need the stamina of a long-distance runner occasionally coupled with the speed of a sprinter.

But detachment, for all its sadness, can also bring a few benefits because there can also be, for some people, a detachment from problems and anxieties, a creating of space between the self and the pressures and demands of daily living. It is ironic that many people go to great lengths to discover ways of disengaging from the world and often spend a lot of money in the process, whilst other people have it thrust upon them without their consent and oblivious of what it may mean to them.

The old biblical image of the rain pouring down day after day and the waters rising, with no end in sight, seems apposite to this situation. And it was here, in the story of the relentless flood, that the rainbow appeared. In the story the rainbow suggests, against all the evidence and challenging their cumulative experience, that there would be a break and that a new day would dawn and the morn would tearless be.

The experience of dementia as a time of fear

Few people make the journey into dementia without a considerable degree of anxiety and fear. Apart from the natural fears associated with losing one's memory and increasing confusion, there are also all the anxieties associated with medical tests and investigations, visits to surgeries and visits from a whole plethora of professionals, often with job titles that are confusing or downright unintelligible to the ordinary person. Within a matter of weeks or months the person is transported from normal everyday living to becoming an object under investigation, very often without being told what the investigators are looking for or whether they have discovered anything. It can be bewildering for the person with dementia and for the carer. There are the additional stresses of getting to the clinics, surgeries or hospitals on time and providing support and encouragement for a person whose confusion is being accelerated by all that is happening to them.

It is a lonely and individual path that has to be travelled. The carer and the person with dementia travel alongside each other, but they do not share the same journey and neither of them knows what lies ahead nor whether they will have the inner resources to meet the challenges ahead.

In terms of finding an image, a story or symbol to hold on to during this time, I find that the struggle of Jesus in the Garden of Gethsemane has certain similarities. He is torn apart by the inner struggle of not knowing what lies ahead, of fearing what it might be and agonizing over the consequences. It is a very personal and lonely struggle and Jesus found that those who were nearest to him, although they wanted to give him all the help that they could, in the end fell away as the desire for sleep overtook them. In the end he was left alone to face his fear and inner turmoil. For many people the anticipation of what might await them is often worse than its actuality. In most situations it is helpful to try to isolate and name the source of our fears. Once they are named it is easier to face them and deal with them. From the general state of fear and anxiety we need to try to break down the individual component parts: once they are isolated, it is often easier to deal with them and, to some extent, neutralize their corrosive influence on our well-being. Then, by looking beyond the wind and rain and focusing upon the rainbow, it might just be possible to believe that the morn shall tearless be.

There is a much loved prayer in the Book of Common Prayer which begins 'Prevent us, O Lord, in all our doings'. 'Prevent us' does not mean stop us, but go before us. 'Go before us, O Lord, in all our doings'...the Christian conviction is that, no matter what fears or terrors lie before us, there is nothing that has not been experienced, in some way, by Jesus. Even through the experience of death we follow in his footsteps. 'Go before us in all our doings with your most gracious favour, and further us with your continual help, that in all our works begun, continued and ended in you'. Begun, continued and ended, our fears and anxieties are experienced within a wider context and, within the invisible fellowship of suffering, we are not alone.

The experience of dementia as a time of despair

Not always, of course, but very often there are moments of utter despair. In religious tradition this is often called the 'dark night of the soul'. It is a time when everything seems to fall apart, when things we thought we could depend upon no longer seem reliable. Jane Williams (1988) describes it in this way:

> It describes a time when we realise that God is bigger than, different from, all our ways of knowing and speaking and praying. It is a time of considerable confusion and fear, when we are unlearning what we thought we knew, but have nothing to put in its place. All the things that seemed so reliable, about ourselves, our place in the world and in relation to God, are no longer certain, we no longer know what weight they will bear and yet, if we cannot lean on them, we do not know how to go forward.

Very often people reach an experience of despair when they no longer feel that they have, or recognize, the resources they need in order to cope. The feeling is heightened by the knowledge that they have to cope. They don't know how to, they feel that they are losing the will to and yet there seem to be no alternatives, no possibilities…nothing. It is a time of despair. For those who stand alongside them there is often little that they can do; they are reduced to silence for they too can see no light ahead; they have no answers, no solutions. But standing alongside is important; perhaps it is the most important thing that they can do. Words are unnecessary; if we find them they are invariably banal or vacuous. There are no words, it is a time to be endured. It is a time when there is no rainbow in the sky, only the relentless rain and the buffeting of the wind.

But this too is part of the Christian tradition, albeit one that is not usually sought after. Williams (1988) continues:

> The dark night of the soul has to be described in negative terms and is experienced as frightening and uncontrolled and yet it is an experience of growth…in the darkness, when we seem to have no knowledge of God at all, in the blankness when our language about God is taken from us, at those times, when God seems least like God, our tradition helps us to know that God is actually breaking in, through the barriers of language and prayer, through the neat models that we have constructed to keep God safe and to harness God for our own use.

Of course, some people do not find a way through their despair and they are sucked into the whirling vortex, sometimes never to escape. But, miraculously, many people do find a way through and they discover that the darkness is not everlasting and that chaos does not reign supreme. It is important that we cling onto that realization and believe that it might be possible for us too.

Donald was dying of cancer and was angry and bitter and in despair, all totally understandable and acceptable emotions, but he wanted to find a way through them. It was suggested that he kept a pencil and paper by his side and that he wrote down the names of all the good people that he had known; that he made a list of memories that were happy and meaningful; that he kept a record of things that he had delighted in. He filled five notebooks and, in the process, found a way through his despair. Everyone is different and will need to find their own particular path, but if we wait long enough, search hard enough or remain open to undisclosed possibilities we may be surprised by the appearance of a rainbow even though the colours may be very faint.

The experience of dementia as a time of pain and heartbreak

Perhaps the most famous sculpture in the world, certainly one of the most famous, is Michelangelo's *Pietà*. It is a marble sculpture showing Mary holding the dead body of Jesus across her lap, just after he had been taken down from the cross. The scene follows one of the most moving pieces of literature where, in the gospels, Mary is described as standing at the foot of the cross witnessing the death of her son. Few things are more heartbreaking than to witness the death of someone who is greatly loved.

Dementia has its own form of heartbreak. It is a painful and difficult journey for the person with dementia as they move into a strange world and it is a different but still painful and heartbreaking journey for those who stand by and watch. It is a pain that cannot be taken away. We cannot inoculate against heartbreak. We have to experience it, endure it and find ways of living creatively with it. In one sense it can never be taken away and it remains with us for the rest of our lives, but in other ways it is possible to find ways of coming to terms with it. One popular hymn puts it this way:

> Hold thou thy cross before my closing eyes
> Shine through the gloom and point me to the skies.

The hymn writer Henry Lyte takes the theme of crucifixion to represent all the pain and heartache we experience and believes that by focusing upon it, it is possible to find a way of moving above or beyond our present situation. It is a different way of saying that we can trace the rainbow and feel that morn shall tearless be. Of course these are both inadequate images but they serve to remind us that, over the years, people have discovered that, despite the reality of their pain, there is the possibility of resolution and of continuing life. It is important that we are honest about the pain and it is important that we recognize that this is a journey which other people have made and their experiences of coming through the nightmare can give us hope at a time of seeming hopelessness.

The experience of dementia as a time of guilt

In John Bunyan's book *The Pilgrim's Progress*, the pilgrim is depicted as travelling with a great bundle tied to his back, weighing him down and causing him distress and tiredness. Later in the book the burden is lifted and he experiences a new-found freedom. It is a compelling image and one which can easily be used to illustrate the experience of guilt. Guilt places a burden upon us, slows us down and tires us out. We never feel free from it until it is lifted. The film *Schindler's List*, about the life of Oskar Schindler, who saved the lives of more than 1200 Jewish people in Nazi Germany, closes with him driving away, being thanked and cheered by the workforce whose lives he had saved. Yet he is full of remorse, saying 'I could have done more, I could have done more' – it is a poignant moment.

Those who care for people with dementia often feel the burden of guilt. It is almost always irrational and unrealistic but this does not diminish the burden. Almost every carer thinks that they could have done more, thinks that they did not care sufficiently or love enough. They punish themselves by setting a standard so high that they are bound to fail. Some carers, of course, could do more and some perhaps did not care sufficiently, but the vast majority are people who endeavour to support and care for people far beyond the call of duty. They give of themselves to an extraordinary extent; they carry the person with dementia along by their love, their care, their perseverance and sheer determination, usually until they can do no more – and they still feel guilty. Feelings of guilt are often intensified when admission into full-time residential care is arranged. The loss experienced by the person with dementia contrasts sharply with the sheer relief of the carer; and there are usually very mixed emotions, which are understandable in the circumstances.

There is no need for those feelings of guilt. Guilt is corrosive and destructive. A friend once said to me that 'your best is always good enough'. Do your best – no one can ask more than that from anyone. Your best may not be enough to cure all ills, solve all problems or heal all hurts, but your best is the most that you have to offer and, once offered, should free you from the burden of guilt.

The seven experiences that I have outlined so far have all been on the negative side, recognizing the pain and distress which is so often experienced by both the carer and the person with dementia. I now want to focus upon four other experiences which, I believe, are also often encountered in this field of dementia care.

The experience of dementia as a time of (re)discovery

'I never knew I could do this until I had to' is a phrase often heard from carers. It could be a man talking about cooking and ironing and delivering personal care or a woman talking about mending fuses, programming the video or handling the household finances. It is a time when traditional gender roles break down and people do whatever is needed to be done, whether they have the experience and background or not. In that way it can be a time of growth and self-realization.

It can also be a time of discovering (or rediscovering) what is actually important in our life or in our relationships. It can focus the mind and help to sort out our priorities. It can also be a time when we discover that we are, in Eileen Shamy's words (1997), 'more than body, brain and breath'.

We may discover these things at the same time as we are experiencing one or several of the more negative aspects mentioned earlier, but they may be the signs of life and seeds of hope that give us the strength to endure and cope with these other things. It is ironic that the experience of dementia can be, at one and the same time, a time of dismantling and also a time of discovery.

The experience of dementia as a time of hope

Just as joy and sorrow are inextricably linked, the one helping to define and illuminate the other, so there can be a relationship between despair and hope. For many people, the experience of despair is the raw material for them hammering out a vision and an understanding of hope. What lies beyond the present impasse? Can there be a new beginning? Does the experience of dementia have to be one of unmitigated gloom and loss or can we discover nuggets of gold, little gems that will feed and nourish us in the future? There is now a considerable amount of recorded experience to suggest that, tragic though the experience may be, it is possible for there to be light and growth, even an awareness that we may trace the rainbow through the rain. It is important that carers and their friends look out for these little signs of hope; they are much needed in the journey through dementia.

The experience of dementia as a time of acceptance

In Shakespeare's *King Lear*, Lear eventually, after scenes of great pathos and sadness, comes to a state of acceptance of his situation and in that acceptance there lies a kind of salvation. Although diminished and stripped of his power he ends the play a more humane and 'whole' person. There comes a time when the fighting must cease and acceptance close in; this does not necessarily have to be seen as a negative development.

Similarly with dementia, it can be very painful, both for the person with dementia and also for the carer, when the time of fighting and struggling gives way to acceptance, but in that act there may also be rays of hope – hope that the struggle and pain and heroic defiance can at last subside and calm can perhaps be allowed to break through. Of course it doesn't always happen like that, but when it does there can be a sense of relief. The violence of the storms pass and the rain appears to be offering hope that the morn might tearless be.

The experience of dementia as a time of mystery

As we endeavour to come to terms with the neurological impediment that manifests itself in whatever form of dementia we are facing, we are invariably moved to reflect upon the amazing complexity and ingenuity of the human brain. It is often only when something goes wrong that we stop for a moment, and realize just how incredible is the human body and the workings of the brain.

For many people it is a time when they stop for a while to consider just what it means to be human. It also raises questions about our understanding of life and death and the meaning of life and the process of dying. We are confronted by a mystery, even more so when we experience, as happens so very often, moments of great clarity amidst all the confusion and forgetfulness.

The experience of dementia can be a time of gratitude

There is a strange relationship between suffering and gratitude. It is almost as though the very experience of suffering helps us to appreciate other things so much more, be they relationships, art, music and literature, creation in all its glory or life itself.

I want to close on a more personal note. Looking back over the last few years I can say in all honesty that having to cope with heart surgery and then, more recently, with cancer has made me realize even more how much I have to be grateful for. There is a sense of wonder about the world when you have journeyed through the cloud of unknowing.

When the person with dementia dies, as we all have to, their death often comes as a source of relief as we recognize that their journey through this strange land has reached its end. There is sadness, of course, both for the person who has died and also for those who have walked alongside them, but there is also gratitude that we have been able to share a little in the mystery, even the majesty, of their life.

We reach a stage in our lives when we have to come to terms with loss and sadness, with pain and suffering, and these are real experiences. But they need to be seen in the context of a wonderful world which gives us so much and which has sustained us over the years. A broken and often tragic world, but a beautiful world none the less.

The rainbow comes to us with a promise of a tearless morn, a morn which may enable us to reflect and be thankful.

Conclusion

An increasing number of people have to address the issue of dementia as they grow older. It is usually experienced as a devastating illness, it is progressive and it is terminal. Without denying the reality of loss and the anxiety and the sadness and grief which is usually associated with such a condition, is it possible to find any signs of hope? I have used the image of the rainbow in this chapter. The rainbow comes to us with a promise of a tearless morn, a morn which may enable us to reflect and be thankful. I do not want to exaggerate the possibilities for hope and I know that many people struggle to find any meaning, any hope when confronted by dementia. On the other hand, I do want to open the door just a tiny bit and suggest that it might be helpful and encouraging to some people if they could take this biblical image and reflect for a while upon its potential for encouragement and sustenance.

CHAPTER 11

Dementia: A Journey Inwards to a Spiritual Self

Christine Bryden and Elizabeth MacKinlay

Introduction (Elizabeth MacKinlay)

We invited Christine to speak at the Centre for Ageing and Pastoral Studies (CAPS) conference in Canberra, and there was some uncertainty as to whether she would be able to speak; her disease was progressing and it was possible that her husband Paul might have to be the speaker. She was ultimately able to come and speak, telling us that this would be one of her last presentations. Speaking publicly was becoming more stressful for her.

I have known Christine for more than a decade. We first met on a Cursillo team in 1995; it was during our preparation for Cursillo that her diagnosis of early Alzheimer's disease was confirmed following extensive investigations and a second medical opinion. She invited me to walk this journey with her into dementia, as I was both a geriatric nurse and a priest. As we met on a regular basis early in her disease, I realized that the way we were able to speak about dementia was unlike any experiences I had previously had as a nurse. As a nurse I had been working out of a medical model of disease, and dementia was 'managed' and in fact, a professional and clinical relationship was maintained between the patient and the nurse, that did not include a mutual journey.

Now I found myself talking with Christine, and listening to her expressing her feelings about having dementia. Christine put this disease right on the agenda for conversation. This grew to become a situation where I could ask her 'How is your dementia?' just as easily as I could ask 'How is your leg today?' of someone who had a fractured femur. This opened up a whole new way of being with people who have dementia.

This chapter consists of the presentation that Christine gave at the conference in Canberra and also another conference she spoke at about a month later, in Berlin. I have set out the whole of her Canberra paper here; the words are too powerful to do otherwise. When I read her second paper, I noted a number of changes in her outlook and concerns, so I have included part of her second paper, only omitting material that appeared in both papers. Christine speaks for herself in the following pages, sharing her struggles and her joys, and the part that her faith has played, and is still playing, in this amazing journey into dementia.

Christine's paper presented at the Canberra CAPS conference

I have no expertise or expert knowledge to offer you, only my personal journey with disability, stigma, and with faith. I was diagnosed with dementia in 1995, and my first book, *Who Will I Be When I Die?* was published in 1998 [under the name Christine Boden]. It reflected my fear of dementia, which was a result of the stereotypical view of this disease causing a loss of self.

Over the years since then I have reflected on my journey of understanding. I can see more clearly who I am now, who I am becoming, and who I will be when I die. Looking back, it has been an amazing journey of self-discovery, change and growth. For me, dementia is a journey to a spiritual self. I have learnt how to dance with dementia, how to adapt to change, how to express my needs, and how to stay in tune with the music as it slows. The title of my second book, *Dancing with Dementia*, tried to capture this positive image of adjustment as I decline. I plan to continue this dance with dementia to my full potential, with my husband Paul alongside me as my dance partner, my care-partner on this journey.

My eleven-year journey since diagnosis with dementia has been like a rollercoaster ride. All sorts of amazing things have happened that I never dreamed were possible. I have battled depression, because of the medical prognosis that was given to me in 1995 – that I would be demented in about five years, and then be in a nursing home for two or three years before dying of dementia.

But I clung to a mustard seed of faith – that I would be able to stay well for longer than expected; be able to help others who had been diagnosed with dementia; and be able to live life to the full. I believed that I was getting better, not as confused, not as slow. Was this because of overcoming depression? Or was it really because the disease process was slowing down, or even stopping? Was this the answer to prayer? But I took a bold step of faith. I went to an introductions agency in 1998 and met, then married Paul. What a rush on the rollercoaster ride!

Not only am I better than I could have hoped for, but I have a loving husband who shares my strong faith and supports me as I decline with dementia. And together we have been able to help others, to advocate nationally and internationally to change the stereotype of dementia, and to work towards hearing the voice of all those who struggle to communicate.

The stereotype of dementia is of the later stages, of the person lacking insight and being unable to speak. The long journey beforehand – between diagnosis and death, of living with dementia each day – is ignored. With the publication of my first book in 1998, I had 'come out'; I felt brave enough to admit to a disease that is feared, and I talked about this long journey with dementia. But I had to battle the stereotype, which had led to the exclusion of people with dementia from many activities, even including those of the Alzheimer's movement. At first, I was not regarded as a credible representative. If I could speak, I did not have dementia.

My diagnosis is still repeatedly questioned. But if I had gone public with, say, a diagnosis of breast cancer, would people want to see the scars? What is it about dementia that makes people demand proof? We applaud the bravery and courage of people battling cancer. Why can't we cheer the dementia survivors? Maybe many of us would survive better and longer, if we did not also have to battle against the stereotype of dementia?

I'm like a swan

I'm like the swan, gliding above the water, paddling frantically beneath the surface. And it feels as if I am paddling faster and faster each day. It seems as if I'm going to sink soon, because the struggle is getting to the point where I feel too exhausted to keep going like this. I can still swim a bit and put on a good show, so that you don't notice much is wrong. Nobody knows, except me and my poor damaged brain, how bad it is. I struggled to write my second book, drawing on speeches, emails, and media interviews, trying very hard to put it all together to make sense. It took six years to finally be able to share my thoughts collectively, slowly, reiteratively, and reflectively. It is an exhausting way to be!

It would be a lot easier for us just to give up, because it is a struggle every day to capture moments of clarity in the fog of our confusion. Unpredictably we can become exhausted, confused, muddle-headed.

Black hole of a life unremembered

Memory comes and goes, so that there are glimpses of past events, or future tasks I wish to do. It's like a 'black hole of a life unremembered'. My memory and my future are captured in a scribble pad that I carry with me. I have a muddle of thoughts, and try to make the most of random bursts of energy and lucidity. This intermittent reception of life as it passes by applies to what I have just asked you too, so sometimes I ask the same question again without realizing I have asked before. I forget the answer, so the question remains to be asked.

I am slowly learning how to live without remembering labels: your name, or even my name. I know faces and know I connect with them somehow, but not why I know them and what I know about them. It is a world in which I know that I know you, but not why I know you. I need many more clues to help me tune in to your recollections of events, and many helpful hints as to who you are so that somewhere along the way I can gain a glimpse of my own shattered memories.

How can we be helped?

The symptoms that we show are the result of several things working together, some of which you can address. Firstly there is the continuing brain damage. A cure to stop and repair this is urgently needed. I hope I last long enough to benefit. Science has reported a cure is five to ten years away for the last ten years; it is ever receding into the future.

While we wait for a cure, you can build on our strengths, working with reminiscence, and most importantly by trying to understand what this assault to our functioning is like. Focus on what we can do, not how we differ from usual levels of capability. There is also plenty you can do to manage our environment, to reduce stress and to interact with us meaningfully in a safe space. The most important way to help is finding out what has given us meaning in our lives. In the face of declining cognition, and increasing emotional sensitivity, spirituality can flourish as an important source of identity.

Reach out to our spiritual self

As time passes, I will need others to understand that my odd behaviour, my lack of social graces, my lack of resources to offer in friendship, do not stem from the soul that lies within me. Rather they are the product of my diseased brain.

The stigma of dementia leads to a view that we are beyond reach of normal spiritual practices. But you can reach out to our true spiritual self that lies beyond cognition and emotion. You can help us to see beyond the transient worldly difficulties of coping each day with brain damage. Find out more about the unique individual who has dementia, about their preferences, and then find ways in which this person can be spiritually nourished. We can find meaning in our spirituality, and you can connect with us, and empower us.

Dementia is often described as a 'loss of self', implying that the person with dementia at some stage loses what it is to be human. But at what stage can you deny me my selfhood? Exactly when do I cease being me? The title of my first book – *Who Will I Be When I Die?* – reflected the fear of losing self, of a future without knowledge of identity. We face this awful fear of ceasing to be, not just a physical death, but also a gradual emotional and psychological death.

The challenge is to live in a world of hope, alternatives, growth and possibility. We need to create a new image of who we are, and who we are becoming. How we do this depends very much on our personality, our life story, our health, our spirituality, and our social environment.

We can choose the attitude we have

I choose to live positively with dementia. In so doing, I am making a journey into the centre of self, away from the complex cognitive outer layer that once defined me, through the jumble and tangle of emotions created through my life experiences, into the centre of my being, into what truly gives me meaning in life.

I've begun to realize that what remains throughout this journey with dementia is what is really important, and what disappears is what is not important. I think that if society could appreciate this, then people with dementia would be respected and treasured. Cognition is like our outer mask, our name, address, job, life story. When we remove this, we find the mask of emotions, of our relationships and feelings. These two masks become faded and scrambled with dementia. But beneath remains the spiritual or transcendent self, which stays intact despite the ravages of dementia. This real self cannot exist independently in our society, which defines people by the outer layers of cognition and emotion, by our masks. It exists in the 'now', continually and eternally.

Like a bud, my true self encapsulates all the potential of what it means to be me. This is a new way of living, maybe even the essence of living, and is the experience of dementia. I have found the answer to the question of my first book: Who will I be when I die? I'm becoming who I really am.

In my journey towards my true spiritual self, with dementia stripping away the masks of cognition and emotion, I'm choosing an attitude of dancing with dementia, and to find out how much dancing is left in me. As each decline becomes apparent, I let my care-partner, Paul, know. Together we adapt to the ever-changing music of dementia. I love the imagery of a couple dancing with dementia. It's a care-partnership, in which we change our steps in this dance, this journey with dementia. I desperately hope for a cure, but in the meantime, I'll try to create and dazzle, despite my limitations. I've done what I can through my books and talks to communicate what it feels like to have dementia and what you can do to help. But time is running out. I feel like a sputtering candle, as it dies down to the last few centimetres of wax. The flame flickers just a bit more brightly before it finally disappears. There is a stream of ideas coming through my brain, yet they don't remain there. They are fleeting glimpses of insight, there one moment, totally gone the next.

Now it is time to rest, and I plan to treasure each moment that remains with my family and my friends. It is time to move away from the bright lights to a corner of the dance floor where the rhythm is slower and the music quieter, but still sweet. All I can do now is sit quietly and listen, and hope for a cure.

Christine's paper presented in Berlin one month later[1]

Originally when I wrote the abstract for this talk, I was going to highlight a few aspects of my book *Dancing with Dementia*, in which I describe what it is like to have dementia and what you can do to help. But since then, I've gone downhill, and this is a more bleak appraisal of where I'm at.

I used to describe living with dementia as a dance of frequently changing steps with my care-partner, my husband Paul. I regarded myself also as a care-partner in that dance, trying to express my own needs, so that he could respond to them as I needed more support, day by day. But the rhythm has changed and I feel more of a care-recipient, rather than an active partner. I am less positive in my daily struggle with decline, as I stumble to the unseen and discordant music of my illness. I am more scrambled, more anxious, more distressed; less able to express my needs, less able to communicate what I am feeling.

This is an inevitable stage of my journey from diagnosis to death, as a younger person with a younger family, and still a vibrant desire to live life to the full. Maybe it is this youthful desire that makes my struggle all the more stressful. I used to be like the swan, gliding above the water, paddling frantically beneath the surface. But after more than ten years of paddling faster and faster each day, now I feel I am sinking, because my struggle with dementia is at the point where I feel too exhausted to keep going like this.

It has been a journey of trauma and recovery from the shock of diagnosis and the horror of the prognosis. The neurologist says I have 'defied specific diagnostic criteria so far', but I don't think I can do this much longer. Now I am too far gone and need to see a new way forward, making the most of family time and trying desperately not to stress everyone out too much, or get too scrambled.

I can't plan, organize or think, but only stress out about muddled events in the past, present and future. There is no structure or pattern to life, just a disjointed stream of sudden stressful surprises and shocks. It would be a lot easier just to give up, because it is a struggle every day to capture moments of clarity in the fog of confusion. Unpredictably I can become exhausted, confused, muddle-headed.

Every moment of the day is a conscious effort. The complexity of so many things is a source of anguish. I feel wretched most of the time, despairing and anxious. My mind is fragmented. I have a muddle of thoughts, and try to make the most of random bursts of energy and lucidity. Stumbling, wobbling and spilling are features of daily life. The world feels like a wobbly place, and it is hard to know where each part of me is in space.

The unreliability of my memory is as if the printer ink is running low and it sometimes works and sometimes doesn't. It is such a hit and miss approach to life. Each day I sink into bed exhausted, worn out from trying to function throughout the day, but I'm so anxious I can't sleep. It feels like I'm on a treadmill spinning out of control. We have reason to be anxious, and we feel out of control. We cannot remember things, so we are always worried that we will lose something. Was there something I promised to do? Was there something I planned to do? These thoughts spin around and get us nowhere, as our mind is a memory blank. Adding to our frustration is our difficulty in communicating – in reading, writing, and speaking. I struggled to write my book, drawing on speeches, emails, and media interviews, trying very hard to put it all together to make sense. And yet many people – including at Alzheimer's Disease International (ADI) conferences – still think there is nothing wrong with me (or my other friends with dementia who speak out), I can't have dementia, simply because I can speak. If only they listened to us, if only they would try to understand us, and appreciate the efforts we make, rather than stand on their medical model!

I could not write that book now, and have no idea how I managed it then. Please read my books and talks, because I did my best to express what this muddle feels like, while I could still get my words together to let you know.

It has been such an effort being public for the last few years, trying to advocate for people with dementia. I first spoke out in Australia in 1999 and at ADI 17 in Christchurch in 2001 (and then at ADI in Barcelona, Santo

Domingo, Kyoto and Istanbul). It has taken a lot out of me. Now I hope to have a little time left to give to my family, and to rest and recuperate enough to enjoy some living at home. I want to be a better wife to my husband while I still can. I want to spend as much time as possible with my three daughters, as they grow to become delightful individual young women. I want to help my husband build his yacht. I have managed to get one more year of travel insurance, so we plan to visit family and friends, overseas and around Australia. Then we must start to plan care options for me, so as to relieve the ever-increasing burden that I am becoming for my family.

If only there was a cure or at least some way to stop the decline, then I could have a little more time. I'm far less positive now, and the dance with dementia has become a wrestle with the ever-pressing presence of illness. I can only choose a positive attitude on those occasions when I see a glimpse of cohesion in my thoughts. The rest of the time it is a stream of fleeting glimpses of thoughts, actions, memories, events. Nothing seems to make much sense unless I desperately try to concentrate.

My story of diagnosis at the age of 46, as a mother of three young girls, and my efforts to live positively, is on the public record. But now my private story continues. This internal tale is one of becoming more stressed, more scrambled, more anxious, and far less capable. I feel that nothing that my caring family do, however hard they try, can ever be enough to compensate for my confusion and wretchedness. But also I feel enormously grateful to them for all their patient efforts. I feel terribly guilty for the increasing strain that my illness is placing upon all of them. What a terrible tension – between never feeling supported enough to cope, and feeling so guilty for all the efforts they have to make for me!

There are no more talks or books in me. I tried my best to communicate what this felt like and what you could do to help. My books and talks are my legacy. Now it's all falling apart. We need to make the most of the years ahead, and make serious plans for my future in care. Paul plans to continue his involvement in the Alzheimer's movement.

My book *Dancing with Dementia* was a huge struggle to write down what I could about the earlier, perhaps more positive part of my journey. I went public at ADI in 2001 with this disease, and have been watched as I struggled to cope with my decline since then. Now I want to move away from the limelight to somewhere more peaceful to be more able to cope with my daily struggles. I want to spend more time with my husband and daughters, and to try to find a way to be a good wife and mother despite my neediness.

I plan to treasure each moment that remains, knowing that time is running out for me, like a candle that flickers as the wax melts down to its last few centimetres. I have done my best to advocate for people with dementia, and have contributed to change. Now I hand this task on to you.

Reflections (Elizabeth MacKinlay)

A hard place to be

Over the last decade Christine has been at the forefront of support and care for people with dementia. She was one of the earliest people with a diagnosis of dementia to take the role of an advocate for others with dementia. As she has explained, this has not been an easy role to carry. The medical model of dementia sets the criteria for dementia and stages of the disease are described. Dementia, in the conventional setting, is 'managed'. Christine has stepped far out from this model and has challenged both professional and community attitudes and beliefs about what is possible for people who have dementia. Yet she still meets opposition, where her very being as a person with dementia is challenged by well-meaning health professionals who do not believe that she can have dementia, simply because she can speak, and further, because she does not fit the stereotype of dementia that the professional textbooks show.

I can have no idea how many people with dementia and their carers Christine has supported and touched in some way. I only can report two instances that I know. One was a couple in Perth who were working with Alzheimer's Association: both the woman with dementia and her husband spoke at a conference I attended. Christine had been inspirational in helping this couple improve their well-being and reach out to others with dementia. The second was a man with vascular dementia whom Christine had supported in writing a booklet for those living with dementia, which we hope will be published and widely distributed.

The place of faith in dementia

It was Christine's faith that first brought us together on this journey into dementia. Through this last decade, it has been her faith that has sustained her. As she finds it increasingly difficult to communicate, it will be her community of faith that will support her. This disease clearly illustrates the interdependency of human beings. While much emphasis is placed on autonomy and self-sufficiency, dementia strips these protective outer shields away and each person with dementia is left vulnerable in a community that values independence, not interdependence. A great strength of Christianity is the community that is possible, worked out through the Body of Christ. We all have need of each other and people with dementia can teach those who do not have dementia what it means to live in the moment and be inspirational in their striving for connection with others. From a faith perspective dementia also provides the opportunity to connect deeply one with another, until late in the disease. At that point, the community of faith becomes the memory and the nourisher of the person with dementia.

The stress of speaking

Paul has been coming with Christine, and speaking more for her, recently. However, this time, Christine was going to speak. When she arrived in Canberra, Christine was very stressed and needed a great deal of support and care, including prayer before she became settled. I remember that I asked her if she would like to attend the conference dinner that evening, and she told me that it would probably be too noisy, and she finds noise very stressing. While recognizing that she was tired and needed to rest, I told her that if she wanted to come, just for the meal and the early part of the dinner, that would be fine. She did come and I watched as she visibly relaxed, to the music provided during the dinner – harp music.

Knowing and its complexities in dementia

Christine's comment 'I know that I know you, but not why I know you' takes us into the complexity of the communication processes of dementia. In one of her earlier publications Christine said that although she may forget the person's name, she still 'knows who you are'. Christine has lost some of her ability to process names and persons, but there is more to knowing than connecting the correct name with the face. In these instances, it could be said that Christine has recognized that she knows, but the specific label seems to have been lost. Some of the work of Damasio (2003) in neurobiology may help explain what is happening for Christine and others who have dementia. Applying tests such as the widely used Mini Mental scale give a fairly crude gauge of cognitive function, but leave much still to be explained about the thoughts, understanding and behaviour of people who live with dementia. According to Damasio, emotions and feelings have complex origins and, working from his theories, I suspect it is likely that aspects of neurobiological functioning are still present and may explain Christine's sense of 'knowing'. At another point Christine remarked 'I need many more clues to help me tune into your recollections of events, and many helpful hints as to who you are, so that somewhere along the way I can gain a glimpse of my own shattered memories.' Christine is developing strategies to deal with her changing cognitive structure to help her to make connections. She said 'I am slowly learning how to live without remembering labels: your name, or even my name. I know faces and know I connect with them somehow, but not why I know them and what I know about them.'

Conclusion

The journey into dementia is a complex and tortuous one. The disease affects not only the person diagnosed, but their family and close friends. Often friends and even family may stop being with, or visiting, the person who has dementia as the disease progresses. Yet, as Christine so clearly shows, it is possible to communicate with people who have dementia. However, we must not allow the disease to get in the way of that communication. Dementia is so widely feared that the mere knowledge of the diagnosis can isolate people from each other. Christine's journey is inspirational and we can learn much from her struggles that will serve to assist us, in developing better means of working with people who have dementia and helping them to improve their quality of life, for as long as possible.

Note

1   I (Elizabeth MacKinlay) have edited this section only to the extent of removing parts that were repeated in both papers.

CHAPTER 12

Bodhi, Karunā and Mettā: Buddhist Perspectives for a Theology of Pastoral Care for the Ageing and Persons with Disabilities

Ruwan Palapathwala

Introduction

While the questions concerning the status of knowledge, its description and who possesses it have received unprecedented attention in the poststructuralist academic literature in the present milieu of postmodernity,[1] the philosophical premises that define knowledge and inform the theological frameworks of pastoral care in the constantly changing religious landscape of contemporary society have received relatively little attention. This is true in pastoral care in general and pastoral care for the ageing and persons with disabilities in particular. As a result, the issues related to the question 'What is holistic care for the ageing and persons with disabilities?' remain either largely unanswered or partially answered and debated among the care-givers ranging from medical personnel, clergy and social workers to politicians and policy-makers to family and friends. In general, with the ageing population[2] and continuing intensification of the pace of life in Western societies, some general trends such as the increased number of residential aged care facilities,[3] intervention projects,[4] and health-care professionals can be noted. To cope with these developments, the institutionalization of age and disability care has emerged as a management strategy in Western market economies. Hence, within institutional and organizational contexts such as the World Health

Organization (WHO), government agencies and the medical profession, the definitions of disability and ageing are limited to a definable understanding of an impairment and deterioration of the physical body which can be measured and assessed for care or management. For instance, according to the definition adopted by the World Health Assembly in May 2001 disability is

> conceptualized as being a multidimensional experience for the person involved. There may be effects on organs or body parts and there may be effects on a person's participation in areas of life. Correspondingly, three dimensions of disability are recognized in International Classification of Functioning (ICF): body structure and function (and impairment thereof), activity (and activity restrictions) and participation (and participation restrictions). The classification also recognizes the role of physical and social environmental factors in affecting disability outcomes. (cited in Parliament of Australia Library 2002)

The 1998 Australian Bureau of Statistics Survey of Disability, Ageing and Carers defined a person with a disability as 'any person with a limitation, restriction or impairment which has lasted, or is likely to last, for at least six months and restricts everyday activities' (Australian Institute of Health and Welfare 1997).

João Pedro Magalhães (2005) defines ageing as 'a progressive deterioration of physiological function, an intrinsic age-related process of loss of viability and increase in vulnerability' and thus a 'complex process composed of several features: 1) an exponential increase in mortality with age; 2) physiological changes that typically lead to a functional decline with age; 3) increased susceptibility to certain disease with age.'

Within the scope of this chapter, I will develop a theology of pastoral care on three premises that can inform the theology and the practice of pastoral care for persons with disability in the later years:

1. that ageing and disability are characteristic of the universal human condition – they are marks of our finitude

2. redemptive compassion

3. the ethic of amity.

This I will do with reference to the Buddhist concepts of *bodhi*, *karunā* and *mettā*.[5] In doing so, I will argue that the efficiency and efficacy of the agencies and personnel that care for older people with disabilities are dependent upon the policies and theological perspectives which are informed and formulated with reference to an understanding of the totality of the human being. The questions related to the totality of the human being – which includes both the physical and spiritual considerations – cannot be adequately addressed without placing them in the context of a religious or philosophical tradition which is formative of the culture in which these questions are asked and addressed. For this reason I have chosen Buddhism as a religio-philosophical tradition to provide the insights to my thesis in the chapter, and I have justified its choice below.

The significance of a religious or a philosophical tradition in this regard is that it provides templates to ask and respond to issues of life concerning the human predicament (the facts of birth, old age, disease, death), and resources necessary to live in spite of the predicament in the here and now; and to evoke hope of overcoming it in the hereafter. Based on an understanding of such concerns a culture forms its worldview and defines its orientation in the world and the destiny of its people (Palapathwala 2006a).

It is in this context that one could appreciate the Christian heritage of the Western civilization. In particular, theological traditions have made an immense contribution to the pastoral theology which has been explicitly and implicitly formative for the church, and also for institutions such as hospitals and for medical endeavours in the Western world. In this chapter I seek to complement the existing pastoral care literature by introducing pastoral perspectives from Buddhism, a religious tradition which is predominantly philosophical and non-thesistic in its orientation when compared with world religions such as Christianity or Islam. With reference to Buddhism I will use the term 'theological' not in the sense of *logos* about *theos*, but rather in the Aristotelian sense of 'the theologic science' of 'being in the highest degree of abstraction' which takes all reality into account and seeks the ultimate and universal causes with a desire to know – *epistēmē* – their ultimate causes. For Aristotle, this knowing then becomes the basis for praxis, the practical sciences of ethics and politics, and for *poiē sis*, the sciences of production, rhetoric and poetics (Lear 1988).

The significance of Buddhism for a theology of pastoral care

The consideration of a pastoral theology with reference to Buddhism is important because, in general, pastoral theology and pastoral care are Christian enterprises that are established exclusively within a biblical understanding of the human person which is framed with reference to God, Christ and his salvific actions and the self-understanding of the church and its mission in the world. This can be demonstrated. According to one of the clearest definitions of pastoral theology it is 'the study of all aspects of the care of persons in the church, in a context of theological inquiry, including implications from other branches of theology' (Lapsley1969, p.43). In a similar vein, pastoral care is defined as 'the practical outworking of the church's concerns for the everyday and ultimate needs of its members and the wider community. That concern has its mainspring in the love that God has for his people, and for his world' (Atkinson and Field 1995, p.78).

Further, the pervasive influence of Buddhism in the world needs to be accounted for – it continues to shape not only the foundations, ethics and attitudes of the cultures of South and Southeast Asia, but increasingly the spiritual landscape of the Western world too. Furthermore, the non-theological resources of Buddhism have the capacity to enrich the already existing Christian theological resources, for interfaith and cross-cultural philosophical perspectives on the question of pastoral care for ageing persons and persons with disabilities.

I have chosen three fundamental Buddhist notions – *bodhi, karuna* and *metta* – to present pastoral theological perspectives on the understanding of the human condition; redemptive compassion for the suffering, and transformative all-embracing-kindness as an art of caring. *Karuna* is selfless compassion that is kindled in one's being for the salvation of all sentient beings as a result of *bodhi* – the awakened knowledge of the true nature of the ill-laden and transient phenomenal world. *Metta* is the emotive and altruistic ethic that enables and facilitates another's happiness and well-being. In Buddhist scriptural literature a distinction is made between the quality of *karuna*: the *karuna* of a fully enlightened Buddha and that of a bodhisatta (Sanskrit: *bodhisattva*, literally meaning 'enlightenment' (*bodhi*) 'being' (*sattva*)). Without necessarily overemphasizing, the compassion of a Buddha is sometimes qualified with the adjective *maha* (great) to highlight the greater capacity of this attribute. However, the *karuna* of a bodhisatta aspirant is seen as one of the perfections which is exhibited, practised and developed mainly by *dana* (generosity), 'though it is also the guiding-star of a bodhisatta's entire career' (Dayal 1932, p.178).

In this chapter I focus on the bodhisatta's compassion because within the Mahāyana schools of Buddhism the prospect of becoming a bodhisatta is prescribed as an ideal to which every human being should aspire. In this way, the bodhisatta ideal presents a model – if not, at least a challenge – for the care-givers to theologize and appraise the fundamental principles that inform the practice of pastoral care.

Three philosophical imperatives in Buddhism

Bodhi *and the universal human condition*

The concept bodhi, from the verbal root budhi, means 'to awaken to understand' and 'enlightenment'.[6] Through *bodhi* 'one awakens from the slumber or stupor (inflicted upon the mind) by the defilements (*kilesa*)[7] to comprehend the Four Noble Truths (*sacca*)' (Commentary to the *Majjhima Nikkaya*, 10, cited in Nyanatiloka 1980, p.72).

According to Buddhism, the Four Noble Truths (*ariyasacca*), as expounded by the Buddha, form the key to comprehension of the universal nature of the human condition[8] which is the prerequisite to wholesome understanding of ageing and disabilities which accompany it. These truths are called 'noble' (*ariya*) because they alone are able to enlighten one about the real condition of the world and thus pave the way to liberation.

The *Dhammacakkapavattana Sutta* (Discourse on the Turning of the Wheel of Law) of the Buddhist Canon contains the Four Noble Truths in their authoritative form and is hailed by the tradition as the *Pathmadhammadesana* – the first preaching of the doctrine – which is the very first public statement of Buddha after his enlightenment. The Four Noble Truths are: *dukkhā* (suffering); the cause or origin of *dukkhā (dukkhāsamudaya)*; the cessation of *dukkha* (*dukkhānirodayā); and the path to the cessation of dukkhā (dukkhanirodhāgaminipatipadā)*. The first two truths deal with the fact and the cause of the human condition, which is a significant part of the condition of the phenomenal world in its entirety – suffering – and the other two truths deal with the remedy for suffering and its cessation. It is recorded in the *Sutta* that Buddha said:

> Now this, O Bhikkhus, is the Noble Truth of *Dukkhā*: Birth is *dukkhā*, ageing is *dukkhā*, sickness is *dukkhā*, dissociation from the loved is *dukkhā*, *not to get what one wants is dukkhā*: in short the five Aggregates (heaps/bundles) resulted/ affected by clinging/attachment are *dukkhā*. There is this Noble Truth of *Dukkhā* : such was the vision, insight, wisdom, knowing and light that arose in me about things not heard before. This Noble Truth must be penetrated by fully understanding *dukkhā* such was the vision, insight, wisdom, knowing and light that arose in me about things not heard before. (*Samyutta Nikā ya*, LVI:11)[9]

As implied in this pronouncement, *dukkhā* can be understood in three ways: first, *dukkhā* as ordinary suffering (*dukkhā-dukkhā): birth, ageing, death, pain, sorrow, grief, lamentation, despair, separation from loved ones, etc.; second, *dukkhā* as *viparināma-dukkhā*, that is suffering caused by change; and third, *dukkhā* as *sankhā ra-dukkhā*. Suffering caused by *sankhāra-dukkhā* means two things: first, suffering caused due to one's existence being intoxicated with false ideas; and second, suffering caused because all phenomena, including one's existence, are conditioned (Boyd 1986). Hence the meanings of the word *dukkhā* are many: difficult to endure, incapable of satisfying, always changing, and incapable of truly fulfilling us or making us happy. It also means unease, unsatisfactory, anxiety, collective-anxiety, physical and emotional pain, and 'ill' in the sense of its use in Old English.

The truth concerning *dukkhā* is neither metaphysical nor an 'absolute' in the sense one may call something a concept, an absolute. In the same way that *dukkhā* is not an absolute, it is also not personal in the sense that one could say 'I suffer'. While the physical and psychological pain one may experience are results of our experience of *dukkhā* it is not the kind of suffering and pain a person, the Devil or even divine-being could inflict upon humanity. It is the truth about the intrinsic value of all phenomena that are subject to change, and therefore impermanent and without any permanent substance. Therefore, all phenomena are stricken with *dukkhā*.

Buddhism explains that the human being is a manifestation of these *dukkhā*-laden phenomena. This means that the human person is made up of a *pañchakhandha*, of five aggregates or five bundles or instruments of clinging: mind and matter (*nama-rūpa*); sensations (*vedana*); perceptions (*saññā*); mental formations (*samkhāra*) and consciousness (*viññana*).

Since the human being is a combination of material manifestation of otherwise independent elements, it is important to note here that in the *Abhidhamma Pitaka* (the Higher Teaching of Buddha) – an erudite compendium of seven books in the Buddhist Canon which deals with the philosophical and psychological aspects of Buddhism – one will not find references to persons or objects such as I, we, he, she, man, woman, tree, lake, etc. Such persons and objects, the writer of the exposition in the *Abhidhamma Pitaka* considers, are relative concepts. Thus, only their ultimate elements are analysed and precisely defined in terms of *khandhas* – the five instruments of clinging to existence – to describe the transient psycho-physical phenomenon which is subject to change and without substance and, therefore, tainted with suffering.

It is only in the general teaching of the nature of these psycho-physical phenomena in the *Suttantā Pitaka* that it is demonstrated how the human being – who is made up of the five instruments of clinging – is ignorant of the true nature of existence and therefore subjects him/herself to birth (*jāt i*), decay and old age (*jarā*), disease (*vyādhi*) and death (*marana*). Hence the description of 'personality' needs to be seen as descriptive of the universal condition of suffering as experienced by the human person who – like all the constituents, the five bundles – is void of substance and a collective phenomenon in constant flux (*santana*). Hence, for one to have a fixation about an ego-centric self – the attachment to the self-idea (*attavadupādā na*) – is both the source and basis of life and suffering in all its forms;[10] it is the pretext to live an ignorant and a delusional life which, in effect, cultivates the conditions (Pali: *kamma*; Sanskrit: *karma*) for the rematerialization of the constituents of the five constituents (*kamma-bhavā* – wrongly understood as reincarnation). Thus the Buddha said of the second Noble Truth:

> Now this, O Bhikkhus, is the Noble Truth of the Cause for *Dukkhā*: it is the craving which produces re-birth, accompanied by passionate clinging (relish and lust), relishing this and that (life): it is the craving for sensual pleasures, craving for being, craving for not-being…This is this Noble Truth of the Origin of *Dukkhā*: such was the vision, insight, wisdom, knowing and light that arose in me about things not heard before. (*Samyutta Nikāya*, LVI:11)[11]

A question that has been raised in the context of attempting to understand ageing and death is the origin of this ill-state of the human condition. In relation to this, in a discourse known as the *Avijjapaccaya Sutta* (Ignorance as a Requisite Condition), Buddha is reported to have refused to answer the question of whether there is anyone or anything lying behind the processes of origin – known as *paticcasamuppāda*, dependent origination. In the discourse Buddha says: 'from ignorance as a requisite condition come fabrications. From birth as a requisite condition, then ageing and death, sorrow, lamentation, pain, distress, and despair come into play. Such is the origination of this entire mass of stress and suffering' (*Samyutta Nikāya*, XII:35). Following the pronouncement, a certain monk asks Buddha the question: 'Which is the ageing and death, Lord, and whose is the ageing and death?' In response to the monk, Buddha says:

> Not a valid question, if one were to ask, 'Which is the ageing and death, and whose is the ageing and death?' and if one were to say, 'Ageing and death are one thing, and the ageing and death are something (or someone else's)', both of them would have the same meaning, even though their words would differ. When one's opinion is that the life-principle (or the soul) is the same as the body and the life-principle is one thing and the body another, there is no holy life. Avoiding these two extremes, the Tathāgata[12] teaches the Dhamma of the middle path: from birth as a requisite condition come ageing and death. (*Samyutta Nikāya*, XII:35)[13]

The remainder of the Noble Truths, the third and the fourth parts, discuss *nibbāna* (*nirvāna* in Sanskrit) and the path leading to *nibbāna*. *Nibbāna* is the state of ultimate release (*vimutti*) from bondage to suffering, the ending of being entangled in the *dukkhā*- laden state of affairs. The path leading to that state is the Eightfold Path which is considered to consist of three-part practical steps: first, ethical conduct – Right Speech, Right Action, Right Livelihood; second, mental development – Right Effort, Right Attentiveness, Right Concentration; and third, wisdom – Right Aspiration and Right Understanding.

The three themes that emerge from this brief discussion are impermanence, suffering, and no-self. In Buddhism these three are known as the three characteristics of existence. The awakening to the knowledge of the source and basis of life and of the universal nature of suffering is considered the most profound and most penetrating knowledge, since it results in three outcomes. It leads the knower to:

1. obtain *nibbāna* and end the turmoil of the five aggregates and thus the rematerialization of the instruments of clinging;

2. cultivate *karunā* (redemptive compassion) for all beings who suffer; and

3. act with *mettā* (all-embracing-kindness) for the well-being of all those who suffer.

Karunā: The redemptive compassion for the suffering

The ethic of compassion in the scriptures of all Buddhist schools is explained with reference to the bodhisatta. Bodhisatta is a person (*satta*) – lay or ordained – who is enlightened or awakened and therefore, while being qualified to attain release (*nibbāna*), out of compassion for the world, renounces it and goes on suffering in *sansāra (the repeated circle of birth and death) for the sake of others. Karunā* is also said to be the word which occurs most frequently in Mahāyana Buddhist texts and thus receives extensive treatment in relation to the *bodhisattva-yana* or the Vehicle of the Bodhisatta. What is distinctive about the bodhisatta ideal in both Theravāda and Mahāyana Buddhism is the superior position which is ascribed to it because a bodhisatta not only attains *nibbāna* but also has the capacity to become a fully enlightened Buddha like Buddha Gotama.[14] The other two paths are known as *Sravaka-yana* and *Pratyekabuddha-yana* – the two paths any person may take according to their ability to pursue *nibbāna*. The *Sravaka* is a disciple of Buddha and the *Pratyekabuddha* is an individual Buddha who attains *nibbāna* alone, at a time when there is no *Samyaksambuddha* (fully enlightened Buddha) in the world.

The other important distinction which is made between these three paths is an important one as it highlights the redemptive or the salvific aspect of *karunā*– the primary motive which gives rise to compassion in the first place. The significance of the redemptive aspect of *karuna* is further emphasized by making a distinction between the degrees of capacity each person on the three paths has to save others by revealing the truth; while the capacity of a *Sravaka* and a *Pratyekabuddha* is limited, a fully enlightened Buddha's capacity is said to be unlimited. Hence the ultimate goal which a bodhisatta cherishes is to eventually become a fully enlightened Buddha. However, while the Pali scriptures of the Theravāda school do not record a single instance of a disciple declaring the aspiration of becoming one, the Theravāda and the Mahāyana schools agree that any person can be a bodhisatta.

Having highlighted the redemptive dimension of *karuna*, the efficacy of the virtue needs to be seen in the context of the Perfections (Sanskrit: *pāramitā*; Pali: *parami*) prescribed in the Buddhist scriptural texts which the bodhisatta aspirants are required to master. The Lotus Sutra of Mahāyana prescribes six Perfections: generosity, morality, patience, effort, meditative concentration and finally wisdom (Dayal 1932).[15] In addition to these, the Theravāda texts prescribe four further Perfections: renunciation, truthfulness, all-embracing-kindness and equanimity. In Chapter IX of *Vishuddhimaggā* (Path of Purification) it is stated that through the development of four sublime or boundless states – all-embracing-kindness, compassion, altruistic joy and eqanimity – one may reach all ten Perfections (Nyanatiloka 1980). In the contexts of all the ten Perfections what is important to note here is the relationship which is being deliberately established between *karuna* and the Perfection of wisdom *(prajñā)* – which is said to be primarily 'to lead the others as a man with eyes leads those who are blind' (Williams 2000, p.134) – and *mettā*. The *prajñā* which is born out of *bodhi* is that 'understanding which sees how it [the phenomenal world] really is in contrast to the way things appear to be' (p.133) and *mettā* is the all-embracing-kindness towards the well-being of all. The fact that *karuna* is listed along with the six or ten other Perfections, and not in isolation, means that its efficacy as a virtue is both affective and effective only within a wholesome framework of the mind.

Thus the proper commencement of the path of the bodhisatta is not a vague sense of wanting to care for others, but 'an actual revolutionary event which occurs in the trainee bodhisatta's mind, an event which is a fundamental switch in orientation from self-concern to concern for others, to compassion'. This motivation is called the 'arising of the Awakening Mind (bodhicitta)' (Williams 2000, p.176) which is then followed by one's taking the Bodhisatta Vows to hasten the achievement of Buddhahood so that one may teach the *Dharma* (the essential nature of things) until all beings have likewise attained release. The Bodhisatta Vows are predominantly Mahāyana in origin and thus various versions of them are also found in Tibetan and Zen Buddhism. In essence, many versions contain a fourfold commitment to save all sentient beings in spite of their innumerability, to extinguish all defilements even though they may be inexhaustible, master all dharmas irrespective of their immeasurability, and to attain enlightenment, in spite of its unsurpassability. These vows too reiterate that the essential motive of *karunā* is soteriological, that is, concerned with the other's redemption from suffering.

Mettā: All-embracing-kindness – the ethic of caring and transformation

The foregoing discussion on compassion has shown that *mettā* (all-embracing-kindness) is one of the ten perfections and also the most important among the four sublime states which facilitates the attainment of all perfections. It is often believed that the true character of the Buddhist ethic is illustrated in this concept of *mettā*. *The term mettā* can also be translated as amity, love, sympathy, friendliness, benevolence and good will. It also means 'emancipation of the heart through love' and 'implies an active interest in [a]nother's welfare' (Law 1986, p.76). In this context, while the 'welfare' of the other is understood in practical terms the well-being of all aspects of life, its ultimate goal, like *karunā*, is salvific.

The idea of *mettā* is the single focus of the Buddhist text, the *Karaniya Mettā Sutta* (The Discourse on All-Embracing-Kindness), which is sometimes also called the 'Hymn of Universal Love'. This sutta is made up of three parts, and underlines the efficacy of *mettā* within a wholesome framework. First, there is the subjective experience, which is the development of the person's own spirituality and the application of all-embracing-kindness in one's day-to-day-living. These three aspects of one's life include the fulfilment of certain virtues (*caritta*) and precepts of abstinence (*varitta*) which are practised through *mettā* and expressed in bodily and verbal action. The virtues expected to be fulfilled are expressed thus: '[the person] should be able, honest and upright, gentle in speech, humble and not conceited, contented and easily satisfied, unburdened and frugal in living, tranquil and calm and wise and skilful, not proud and demanding in nature'. And the precepts of abstinence are expressed thus: 'also, let the person not do the slightest thing the wise would later reprove' (*Sutta Nipatta*, 1:8).[16]

Second, there is the development of all-embracing-kindness as a distinct technique of meditation leading to higher consciousness induced by absorption (*samadhi*). The stanza expresses it thus:

> Whatever living creatures there be, whether they are weak or strong, omitting none, the great or the mighty, medium, short or small, the visible and the

invisible, those living near and far away, those born and to-be-born – may all beings be at ease, let none deceive another, or despise any being in any state, let none through anger or ill-will wish harm upon another. (*Sutta Nipatta*, 1:8)[17]

The Sanskrit word for *mettā* is *maitri̱ and in the Hindu scriptural texts one finds that maitri̱* is the state of a *mitra*, a friend. Hence, 'a friend is one who shows love (*mettā yati*), produces love (*mettim paccutthapeti*), and also cherishes affection (*sineham karoti*) towards others' (*Jatakā*, I:365, cited in Law 1986, p.76).

Third, there is the cultivation of an unreserved commitment to the philosophy of universal love, which is extended through all bodily, verbal and mental activities to personal, social and other dimensions of life. In the stanza it is expressed thus:

Even as a mother protects her child with her life, so with a boundless heart should one cherish all living beings; radiating kindness, in all its height, depth and breadth, all throughout the universe; free from hatred and ill-will, whether standing or walking, seated or lying down; free from drowsiness, one should sustain this recollection. This is the sublime abiding. By not holding to fixed views, the pure-hearted one, having clarity of vision, being freed from all sensual desires, is not born again into this world. (*Sutta Nipatta*, 1:8)[18]

The ultimate goal of *mettā* – the altruistic wish which leads to transformative action to free another from suffering – is clearly expressed at the conclusion of the stanza: 'may all be well and secure, may all beings be happy!'

A practical device, that has been developed since the early days of Buddhist practice, for everyone who seeks to cultivate the transformative ethic of *mettā*, is known as *mettā -bhavanā*, the meditation on universal love. Based on canonical and commentarial sources, there are three specific modes of meditation.[19] Since Buddhist cosmogony places existence on earth in the context of numberless world-systems that are inhabited by infinitely varied categories of beings in different stages of evolution, the three types of meditation are based on three modes of radiating boundless universal love. The three modes of meditation are generalized radiation (*anodhiso-pharana*), specified radiation (*odhiso-pharana*), and directional radiation (*disa-pharana*). Respectively, each mode of meditation wishes redemption from all ill, and happiness to: all beings; specific beings such as females, males, noble ones and gods, etc.; and beings dwelling in all directions such as the north and south and so on.

Furthermore, the redemptive aspect of *mettā* can be seen in its use as a spiritual formula – a *paritta* – that is capable of providing one with protection from ill and healing from diseases. Hence, in Buddhist countries the recitation of *paritta* for the sick is a common practice.

A Buddhist–Christian theology of pastoral care

Within the non-theistic threefold Buddhist framework of *bodhi*, *karunā* and *mettā*, I have discussed the teaching that one's knowledge of the universal human condition gives rise to redemptive compassion, and becomes an enabling force of transformative care, which is also liberative. In many respects, this knowledge and compassion are interrelated; without these, caring will be neither transformative nor redemptive, but pity-driven or obligational, if the motive for caring is not evoked by compassion. Compassion will not be redemptive, but mere goodness and sentimentality, if one's understanding of the essential nature of all phenomena has not given birth to it. In the same way, knowledge about the human condition will not be knowledge if it has not risen out of *bodhi*; it is knowledge only if its logical outcome moves one to compassion with a determination to alleviate the suffering of all beings, and care for all beings with an all-encompassing-kindness until their redemption is realized. In these ways, the Buddhist religio-philosophical system's profound insight into human existence and its essentially soteriological ideology have many contributions to make to pastoral theology in general and with regard to the care of the ageing and persons with disabilities in later life in particular. While the implications of the issues discussed below need extensive treatment elsewhere, the outlining of three major contributions of Buddhism to pastoral theology – conceptual or theoretical, analytical and practical – will suffice for the purposes of this chapter.

The theoretical contribution of Buddhism to pastoral theology

When Christian theological frameworks and the Buddhist conceptual frameworks that may be applied to a discussion on the human condition, compassion and caring are compared, significant differences are to be noted. While Christian pastoral theology addresses the issues of human frailty, the particular Buddhist contribution to theology is its detailed description of the human condition outside the Creator/creature, Divine/human and sin/forgiveness frameworks. In many respects, the exposition of the grounds for redemptive compassion and the virtues of the bodhisattas – novices and accomplished ones – that also exemplify the desired character and stature of a care-giver, are important contributions to Christian pastoral theology. In this regard, it must be noted that the idea that a bodhisatta is a human being who suspends their own liberation to intervene in the affairs of suffering humanity constitutes a Buddhist doctrine of grace. Thus the Buddhist idea of compassion provides pastoral theology with insights into the possibility of the care-giver's being an embodiment of grace. Buddhism signifies this possibility without reference to a sacramental theology or a doctrine such as the Pauline idea of justification through faith by grace. The Buddhist idea of all-embracing-kindness is also of great importance to Christian pastoral theology. While the Christian notion of *agapē* signifies a profound understanding of unconditional love for the other, a comprehensive understanding of its implications presupposes an *a priori* knowledge of God's unfathomable love, whereas *mettā* is not dependent upon *a priori* knowledge of Divine love; it presupposes knowledge about the essential nature of all phenomena.

These notable differences need to be seen not as contradictory but as complementary; for the fundamental issues they deal with – the human condition, compassion and caring – cannot be essentially different realities. What is different is the mode of analysis and conceptualization. In that respect, the Buddhist perspectives which have been discussed here have a significant interfaith contribution to make to contemporary pastoral theology in general.

The analytical contribution of Buddhism to pastoral theology

The particular analytical contribution of Buddhism to pastoral theology needs to be seen with regard to the contextualization of pastoral care for older people in contemporary society in general, and in the developed world in particular. In general, the concern here is the broader context in which the issues of ageing and disabilities need to be analysed and discussed for consideration in pastoral theology.

The first issue is the negative attitude toward old age and accompanying disabilities in contemporary society. Owing to this, not only is the word 'old' made to carry a pejorative sound, but also attempts are made on the grounds of 'political correctness' to avoid the word when referring to people of advanced years. As a result, the 'aged' are referred to in other ways: 'senior citizens', 'golden-agers', 'elderly persons', 'persons in the harvest years' and so on (Papalia and Olds 1992, p. 472). While these terms also attempt to address the sensitivity related to discrimination based on age – ageism – nevertheless, they also genuinely assist in avoiding the images the word 'old' brings to mind: feebleness, incompetence, and narrow-mindedness (p.472). However, since the myth of 'youth' has fascinated human beings of all cultures both old and new, the two other issues of consumerism and commodification of ageing need to be seen as the sinister issues that have made the contextualization of pastoral care for the ageing difficult. While consumerism has made ageing a defined market category for profit, commodification of ageing people has invented new life-course vocabularies that reconstruct maturity, ageing, life-course, senior citizenry, masculinity, femininity, sexuality and ageing bodies. These reconstructions have enabled the market and lifestyle industries to create an idealized culture of 'ageless' consumers and active populations. Accessory to these trends is also the new concept of sexual 'function' which has emerged as a significant concern to rehabilitate the ageing body for lifelong sex and successful lifestyles (Katz and Marshall 2003).

Lunsford and Burnett (1992, p.56) argue that the 'new age elderly' have a 'cognitive age younger than their chronological age' as a possible reason for these developments in the commodity market. My interpretation is that the 'cognitive age' here refers not to the health of one's mental capacities – that is, 'being young at heart' – but to an unhealthy attitude of being younger than one really is, which is then outwardly expressed through dress, lifestyles and behaviour patterns which are naturally not conducive to, and are at odds with, one's age and maturity. While the increasing health and fitness consciousness in the contemporary mindset of many can contribute to one's having a physical age younger than one's chronological age and is a desirable advantage for the ageing, the unhealthy attitude of being younger is both unsound and tragic. It is unsound because such an attitude could be psychologically detrimental to one's well-being as the ageing process continues to its natural end. It is tragic because it is a denial of the greatness of a complete life-cycle in the natural order of the human life process.

The Buddhist analysis of the human phenomenon in the context of the Four Noble Truths is a complete antithesis to the consumerist and commodified notion of age. Buddhism, with its fundamental engagement with *dukkhā*, keeps the stark reality of suffering in perspective. It leads one not to denial but to an encounter with the noble truth of suffering, in which alone lies the true meaning of existence and the possibility of victory over its vicissitudes and temporality. While the evaluation of each experience may differ, if understood properly, it assists one to both value and understand old age (*jara*) as but one aspect with equal standing with infancy, childhood and youth which are also without permanency and in continuous flux. That is to say that in redemption – the spiritual state of nibbāna or when God has wiped every tear from our eyes (Revelation 7:17), the state in which the turmoil of physical existence has ended – the temporary and age-defined value of infancy, childhood, youth and old age will have ceased to have any meaning. Thus, the denial of ageing and disabilities is not only a psycho-physical handicap in the everyday affairs of life but also an impediment to one's spiritual advancement and one's ultimate redemption.

The contribution of Buddhism to practical pastoral theology

The particular practical contribution of Buddhism to pastoral theology needs to be appreciated in the practical circumstances of debilitating old age and all its consequences which care-givers – medical personnel, clergy, chaplains, social workers, families and friends – confront in real life. In this respect, pastoral theology deals with the psychological and physical feebleness, incompetence and illness experienced by ageing people, and concerns itself with four practical issues:

1. the 'hands-on' caring for the persons who are ageing with accompanying disabilities;

2. meeting the spiritual needs of ageing people;

3. meeting the spiritual needs of the loved ones of the ageing; and

4. the carer's spirituality and their reconciliation with the 'unacceptable' – ageing and disability.

The unique contribution of Buddhism to these four areas of concern in pastoral theology is found in the principal notion of *bodhi* – the knowledge of the universal human condition – which is then expressed in practical terms through the two virtues of *karunā* and *mettā*. As discussed above, if seen in isolation, these two virtues have neither meaning nor efficacy. *Karunā* and *mettā* were said to originate out of *bodhi* which, in effect, cultivates compassion and loving-kindness in a person, with an urge to free all beings that suffer and facilitate their happiness and well-being. Even though the bodhisatta may be seen as an embodiment of grace and thus an external agency that intervenes in enabling redemption, other than paving the way for one's release through understanding (the Four Noble Truths), the bodhisatta does not, and cannot, offer salvation. Through these three interrelated Buddhist notions, Buddhism makes its contribution to the aforementioned four practical concerns of pastoral theology.

Subjectively and objectively, *mettā* facilitates the 'hands-on' caring of ageing persons. Subjectively, it prepares and qualifies care-givers to selflessly apply themselves in the service of the person. In practical terms, even when the carer is employed, the *mettā*-driven caring is not proportionate to the remuneration of the carer, but rather proportionate to the degree of understanding the carer has of both their own and the care-receiver's share in the human condition. Objectively, *mettā*-driven caring seeks to extend one's knowledge and wish for the other's welfare in two directions: first, to the care-receiver. When it is physically possible, this happens through allowing a reciprocal understanding of ageing and disability to develop between the care-giver and the care-receiver.

It is at this point that the spirituality of the care-receiver is cultivated and facilitated by the carer, to accept the circumstances of ageing with the acceptance of the caring exemplified by the carer. Second, $mett\bar{a}$-driven caring enables care-givers to extend their understanding to the socio-political dimensions of caring, and thus influence and lobby for better policies and health care for ageing people.

The virtue of $karun\bar{a}$ makes a unique contribution to the last two above mentioned concerns of practical theology: meeting the spiritual needs of the loved ones of older people and those of the care-giver. As demonstrated, the cultivation of the Buddhist ethic of compassion is subjected to one's awakening to the essential nature of the phenomenal world. This entails not only one's acceptence of the unacceptable – ageing and disability – which is characteristic of all things which are transient and without substance and thus is tainted with suffering – but also a resolution on one's part to share this understanding with others. One's acceptance of the unacceptable is also one's acceptance of one's heritage in the human condition. This acceptance facilitates the harnessing of the spirituality of the care-givers which enables them to accept themselves in solidarity with all who suffer. It is such a spirituality which empowers one to participate in the caring of the wider communities associated with ageing. Hence the Buddhist notion of $karun\bar{a}$ makes a distinctive contribution to pastoral theology in underlining the dynamic and redemptive bodhisatta ethic that is vital in the character of the care-givers and in their act of care-giving.

Conclusion

The global consciousness which is an essential ingredient of the twenty-first century requires that, besides technology and medical sciences, faith and religious traditions engage in a fruitful dialogue to address fundamental experiences that characterize human existence. Birth, ageing and death are among such fundamental experiences that require an ongoing understanding, so that the suffering which accompanies those experiences may be alleviated with compassionate caring. In this respect, Buddhism has a significant contribution to make to Christian pastoral theology and vice versa. The uniqueness of Buddhism's contribution in this regard is its non-theistic but non-humanist religio-philosophical system which expounds the human predicament, and, like Christianity, with salvation as its ultimate gift to humanity. The uniqueness of Christianity's contribution is its theistic system which theologically elucidates the human predicament, and, like Buddhism, its ultimate gift to humanity. In these regards, together in dialogue, both Buddhism and Christianity have a significant contribution to make to the field of pastoral theology.

The common gift of salvation challenges Christian pastoral theology on another frontier: not only to be informed by Buddhist perspectives on pastoral care, but also to traverse, in partnership with Buddhist philosophy, previously unexplored grounds to inquire what essentially constitutes suffering and redemption. Without such interfaith understanding and respect for one another's enlightening perspectives, the depth of caring we attempt to espouse in a religiously diverse and technologically sophisticated world may face the risk of becoming another consumer-specific commodity that is serviced – out of charity or for profit – for the ageing and their disabilities in later years.

Notes

1   A major representative of this line of thought is Jacques Derrida. In his own particular poststructuralist blend of philosophy, linguistics, and literary analysis which is applied to Western forms of knowledge (e.g. humanities, science, philosophy) he deconstructs the assumed 'centres' and 'origins' upon which they have built themselves up. According to Derrida, these centres and origins have no basis in reality – they are only myths. See Derrida 1976.

2   According to the Australian Bureau of Statistics, one in five people in Australia (3,958,300 or 20.0%) had a reported disability, and there were 3.35 million people aged 60 years and over (17% of the population), which compares to 3.0 million people (16%) in 1998. In 2003, just over half (51%) had a reported disability, and 19 per cent had a profound or severe core-activity limitation (Australian Bureau of Statistics 2004c).

3   See, for example, Australian Institute of Health and Welfare 2000b.

4   See the Australian Government's final report on the National Evaluation of the Aged Care Innovative Pool Dementia Pilot project (Hales, Ross and Ryan 2006).

5   The Buddhist words used in this chapter are in Pali.

6   In Sanskrit *bodhi* means the 'intellect' – the 'higher mental faculty, the instrument of knowledge, discernment, and decision' – and while it is understood with slight variations in different philosophical systems, in general it is contrasted 'with *manas*, mind, whose province is ordinary consciousness and the connection of *atman* (spirit) with the senses'. It is, however, 'a higher faculty that acts in sense percepts organized by *manas* and furnishes intellectual discrimination, determination, reason, and will' and 'is at the very core of one's being, as a sentient creature , and the closest mental faculty to the *atman*, real Self or spirit' (Bowker 1997, p. 171).

7   The *Vishuddhimaggā* (Path of Purification) – the fifth-century CE scholastic Pali compendium of Buddhaghosa – refers to the defilements as mind-- defiling unwholesome qualities and lists ten such qualities: greed (*lobhā*), hate *(dosā)*, delusion *(mohā)*, conceit *(manā)*, speculative views (*ditthi*), sceptical doubt

(*vicikicchā*), mental torpor (*thīna*), restlessness (*uddhaccā*), shamelessness (*ahirika*), and unconscientiousness (*anottappa*) (Nānamoli 1979, pp.49,65).

8 The Buddhist theory of knowledge explains that what Buddha had was a threefold knowledge (*tisso vijja*) consisting of retrocognition (*pubbe-nivasanussati*), clairvoyance (*dibba-cakkhu*) and knowledge of the destruction of defiling impulses (*asvakkhaya*) which are classified under what is known as *abhiñña* – the six higher powers. *Abhiñña* means the 'comprehension achieved on attainment of the paths and fruitions'. Such knowledge is known as *bodhi* – awakened to understand. It is important to note that retrocognition (*pubbe-nivasanussati*), clairvoyance (*dibba-cakkhu*) and the knowledge of the destruction of defiling impulses (*asvakkhaya*) do not mean some magical power. In the Buddhist context they mean the 'divine eye' which is awoken so that one may see causes (one's own former existences and decease and survival of beings) and the causal process with regard to the defiling impulses. See Kalupahana 1976 and Jayatilake 1963.

9 The translation is mine.

10 For a detailed discussion on the question of self see Palapathwala 2006b.

11 The translation is mine.

12 Tathāgata means 'Perfect One' – an epithet of the Buddha used by him when referring to himself.

13 The translation is mine.

14 In the Theravāda Pali Canon the term bodhisatta was used by Buddha to refer to himself in his previous lives before he was enlightened.

15 Another late Māhayana sutra known as *Dasabhumika* (Ten Stages) lists another four perfections: skilful means, resolution, spiritual power and knowledge (*jñana* – knowledge – in addition to *prajñā*, wisdom).

16 The translation is mine.

17 The translation is mine.

18 The translation is mine.

19 For detailed information on instructions on the theory and practice of *mettā-bhavanā* see *Visuddhimaggā*, Chapter IX.

CHAPTER 13

'Who is God in the Pit of Ashes?': The Interplay of Faith and Depression in Later Life

Dagmar Ceramidas

Depression affects about 17 per cent of community-dwelling Australians over 65 years of age (Looi 2005). Although the disease is easily treatable, it is believed (Jorm *et al.* 2004; O'Connor, Rosewarne and Bruce 2001) that less that 50 per cent of older depressed people seek treatment for depression. Lack of diagnosis of depression can result in reduced quality of life physically and spiritually as the person struggles to cope with everyday activities. It can also lead to self-harm, particularly for males over 75 years of age, who are in the highest risk category for suicide across all age groups (Trewin 2004).

This chapter offers some findings from a recent study into the interaction between Christian faith and depression in the later years of life. Findings are revealed through participants discussing the challenges of depression against their background of faith, reflecting on their church's response to their illness, and through exposing some personal beliefs that negatively impacted on participants' faith during depression.

Within this chapter, depression is viewed from a spiritual perspective complementing existing knowledge of the bio-psycho-social models accepted in general medicine (Kaplan and Sadock 1991). Some spiritual aspects of depression are presented, together with suggestions for pastoral care of elderly Christian people through and between episodes of depression. The study findings can be applied generally to other faiths and community groups.

Depression in the Australian community

In Australia in 1997, depression requiring medical intervention had a prevalence of one in four (Australian Bureau of Statistics 1998). This includes about three in every 25 community-dwelling Australians over 65 years of age. A 2001 survey of Australians living in residential care revealed that 'between 40% and 60% of high care residents and 25% to 51% of low care residents are depressed' (Fleming 2001b). In 2005, 13.1 per cent of Australia's population was over 65 years (Australian Bureau of Statistics 2004b) and the proportion is projected to increase to between 29 per cent and 32 per cent by 2101 (Australian Bureau of Statistics 2004a). It is therefore timely to consider and plan for nurturing those aspects of a person's life that have greater impact on well-being and quality of life in the later years. The benefits of thorough early planning will be evident in subsequent years when the burden of ageing on the Australian economy is expected to increase (Commonwealth of Australia 2002).

There is now sufficient research to suggest that healthier ageing is related to increased religious activity (De Leo 2002; George *et al.* 2004; Idler 2004; Koenig *et al.* 1997; Krause 2003), and that elderly people who have an inner spirituality derive security, a sense of belonging and connectedness through their active belief in God (Kaldor, Bellamy and Powell 1997; Kaldor, Dixon and Powell 1999; Kehn 1995; Levin and Taylor 1997; McFadden 1996; Rudin 2006). But it is not merely 'religious activity' that makes the difference. Rather, the individual meaning of and motivation underlying each activity have been revealed as critical factors in the positive benefits of religious involvement (Diener and Clifton 2002; Dudley and Koder 2002; Moberg 2005).

The study

My doctoral study explored Christian faith in the later years of life. Specifically, the study explored meaning attributed to faith-related behaviours and the effect of these behaviours in the lives of elderly Christian people who suffer depression. For logistical reasons, the study focused only on the Christian faith.

The study used grounded theory, which may be defined as the generation or creation of sociological theory based upon data systematically obtained from social research (Charmaz 2003; Glaser and Strauss 1967). New data build on previous information to enrich and generate an evolving sociological theory grounded in participant experience.

Grounded theory was chosen because it allows open inquiry into the social and emotional factors embedded within personal meanings of faith-related behaviours for individuals. Among other things, motivational, historical, social, cultural and individual factors are likely to influence a person's acceptance of and participation in faith-related behaviours. These factors and behaviours can be captured for analysis through grounded theory methods. Further, any discussion of faith involves emotions, potential stigma, and intimate perceptions, none of which can be measured quantitatively (Stoneking 2003) and all of which beg exploration through the use of grounded theory.

This study comprised 20 participants over 65 years of age who self-nominated as people of Christian faith and had experienced depression or severe loneliness. Following informed consent, each participant completed the brief 15-item Geriatric Depression Scale (GDS) (Yesavage *et al.* 1983) and a semi-structured interview of between one and two hours in length. All participant interviews were recorded and transcribed prior to importation into the NVivo (Richards 2002) software package for coding. Following coding, analysis and cross-referencing allowed the identification of themes arising from the participant interviews. These themes were then examined for interrelationships and against the research questions.

The GDS and the international diagnostic tool, the Diagnostic and Statistical Manual of Mental Disorders version 4 (DSM-IV) (American Psychiatric Association 1994), were used to ascertain the group's homogeneity with respect to depression.

Same black dog, different tale

All participants but one (n=19) in this study experienced depressed mood as described in criterion A and met criteria B–E inclusive, as listed in the DSM-IV for Major Depression or Major Depressive Episode (p.327). Eighty-five per cent of participants had been diagnosed by a medical practitioner or psychiatrist and 75 per cent were using medication at the time of interview. An additional 15 per cent of participants had declined medication. Four participants had been hospitalized for depression; and a further four reported that hospitalization had been suggested but was declined for various reasons. Seventy-five per cent of participants had multi-episodic depression throughout their lives.

More than half of the participants had contemplated suicide, and 20 per cent of these had made serious plans or an attempt. Seven of this group gave family reasons for not acting on their plans and six attributed their inaction to their belief in God. One participant said

> Even though there was a sort of breakdown in relationship [with God during the depression], I think if I didn't have that belief system, there wouldn't have been much there even when I stabilized... I might have done more than

contemplate suicide as a solution. But having the belief system, having the relationship with God just enabled the stabilization...it enabled me to see new directions in life, where old doors had closed. (David)

The tales unfold

Eighty per cent of participants described a lifelong relationship with God. Two participants had chosen Christianity in mid-life but retrospectively recognized that God had been 'overseeing' their lives despite their lack of earlier acceptance of faith. The study findings suggested no positive differences in depression for participants whose stories expressed greater frequency of prayer, of church attendance, involvement in Bible studies or participation in fellowship groups. This is consistent with literature wherein Shulik (1992) and Coleman *et al.* (2002) found that people who have either high or low faith are more likely to experience greater depression than people whose faith is uncertain.

With respect to levels of faith, it became evident that while all participants claimed to have a relationship with God, the quality of this relationship varied among participants. Participants who spoke about God as a close friend, chatting with Him 'just because He's there', seeking His involvement in decision-making and everyday events of their lives, were allocated to the *close group* (11 participants). Participants who described God as more of an acquaintance than a close, personal friend were allocated to the *distant group* (9 participants). It was not clear how these differences in quality of relationship with God came about particularly as depression appeared to be more severe for close-group participants.

The critical factor in religious involvement leading to improved well-being is not so much the presence of faith-related behaviours but more the underlying motivation. Participants' stages of faith development were explored to provide better understanding of the motivation underlying their faith-related behaviours.

The majority of models of faith development were developed for religious education (Cooke 2001; Lake-Smith 2006; Ziettlow 2004) and hence were limited to three or four stages that ended in early adulthood. Fowler's model (Fowler 1981), while 'not descriptive of Christian faith development' (Jones 2004) and 'allow[ing] for a variety of traditions, Christian and other' (Macleod 2005), offers six stages of faith development and provides thorough descriptions at each stage, permitting more confident determination of participant levels of faith development. Cooke's model was used as a comparison because it continued beyond adolescence and, being grounded in an applied faith perspective, offered an alternate paradigm.

Comparing the close and distant groups against both Fowler's and Cooke's stages of faith development revealed that the faith development of distant-group participants had arrested at earlier stages of life, while the faith development of close-group participants had progressed further.

Fowler acknowledges that it is common for faith development to 'arrest' (1981, pp.50–1) and remain at a particular stage, usually midway in the six-stage process. None of the distant participants had progressed on their faith journeys beyond Fowler's stage four; however, all close participants were in stages five or six of Fowler's faith model and the highest stage of Cooke's model. The study revealed a relationship between level of faith development, closeness of relationship with God and motivational factors underlying faith-related behaviours. Participants who demonstrated internal motivation underlying their faith-related behaviours had advanced further on their faith journeys and had a more intimate relationship with God – but appeared to have more severe depressive episodes.

Faith applied

A factor present to close participants but missing in distant participants was that those who on reflection had applied Romans 8:28[1] in their lives had been able to progress on their faith journey. Through their faith journey, some participants had experienced that 'God brings men into deep waters, not to drown them, but to cleanse them' (John Aughey).[2] The close group were able to view depression in a positive light, while the distant group did not recognize any positive outcomes arising through depressive episodes, seeing them only as impositions on their lives. The close group reported being overall more satisfied with their lives.

A level of transcendence was therefore operating in the lives of the close-group participants. Despite the storms of depression and other potentially negative factors in their lives, participants with a closer relationship with God were to some degree able to traverse and rise above the circumstances that might otherwise have resulted in greater debilitation.

The interplay of faith and depression
Negative effects of depression on faith

All participants found that depression tested their faith and subsequently their relationship with God. Participants struggled to find God's presence during depression, hence they began to doubt their faith and sometimes even God's existence. *Knowledge* of the promise of God's unfailing presence didn't quench the agonizing *feelings* of the perception of being disconnected from God or abandoned by Him. For some participants, this disconnection was devastating and resulted in thoughts of self-harm as the only option to life in a Godless world.

For many participants, the debate between head knowledge versus their experienced feelings looped continuously in their minds, each iteration increasing their sense of hopelessness and despair. While some participants were able to verbalize God's promise, 'I will never leave you or forsake you' (Hebrews 13:5), their 'pit of ashes' *feelings* were not eased by this scripture, resulting in expressions of self-blame such as the following:

> Well, I feel that it's my fault. I feel God is there, but I'm just not producing whatever it is that you need to produce to draw close to Him to get His help… But now I'm so depressed I'm incapable of doing things and I feel worthless doing it and I feel that I've let God down. I never feel the other way. I never feel that God's let *me* down, because I don't think that He would. Now *I've* got to find a way. (Elliot)

Although some participants expressed anger at God when a depressive episode took hold, such expressions demonstrated participants' vital need to remain connected with God, regardless of the situation. The duration of the anger varied among participants who in retrospect sought forgiveness from God, recognizing the anger as part of the experience of depression.

Again speaking on behalf of some participants, a qualified and appointed chaplain expressed that depression 'fed into this whole dynamic for me, which I found very scary. I mean, it really is basically saying…not what *is* God, but *is* there a God?' As a result of depression, this participant from the distant group came to doubt the very essence of her lifelong faith and resolved to leave the church. Repeated episodes of depression were life-changing for this participant.

Where faith was built during and despite depression

Even upon reflection, distant participants could not see positive outcomes of depressive episodes in the broader expanse of their lives and were more prone to impetuous action during an episode, an action that was at times regretted post facto. Conversely, close-group participants came to view depression as a recurring 'blip' on the horizon of their lives but anticipated positive outcomes from each episode. This increased their faith as they recognized that 'God meant it for good' (Jeremiah 29:11) and was in fact loving them despite their illness.

One close-group participant heard God's voice through her depression, 'But all the while God was saying "I'm in charge here. You let me run the ship; you just be a guest on my ship."' While struggling to overcome her thoughts and feelings of desperation, this participant forced herself to rely on her knowledge of the scriptures, the image she had built of God's character and her relationship with Him. 'And that was the only thing I could do, was to look to God and believe that He was in charge, that He had the boat, that...I was to be a cruise passenger.'

Close participants illustrated how their faith allowed them to positively reframe depression. One participant thanked God for allowing her to 'exercise my spiritual muscles', likening the depressive episode to a 'spiritual gym'. Participants whose strategy was to keep busy during depression believed that depressive episodes were God's way of forcing them to rest. Some male participants considered that a depressive episode was God's way of catching their attention, enabling them to review and renew their lives.

Several participants drew on their knowledge of the scriptures to affirm God's love and abiding presence for them. In combining the words of Scripture with their understanding of God's character, these close-group participants realized a degree of victory over their depressive feelings and used this realization to 'move forward' – even if moving forward simply constituted the ability to not struggle but 'to be still' and in God's presence during depression. Participants with a distant relationship with God had not developed enabling images of God's character hence were unable to reach this point of resting or surrender during depression. Positive outcomes of faith on depression were seldom evident for distant-group participants.

Is Christianity a hindrance or a help? Negative effects of 'faith' on depression

Some common features of depression are: faulty thinking, negative thinking patterns and the habit of perceiving positive or neutral events as negative (Beck 1967). For some participants, faith seemed to worsen the depression as their minds replayed negative thoughts and beliefs that were discovered to be unfounded and unscriptural (Ellison 1994; Moriarty 2006). Following counselling that exposed and rectified their misunderstandings (Anderson 1990, 1993; Close 2000; Doogue and Sturgess 2005; Snyder, Sigmon and Feldman 2002), these participants were released from the captivity of such confounding thoughts.

Some participants believed the depression was their 'fault' and subsequently blamed themselves for 'being in this Godless place'. The resulting guilt exacerbated their depression. Theologically, the Bible clearly states that Jesus' life was given to atone for all sins of all people (Romans 3:25; Hebrews 2:17), and is replete with examples of Jesus' forgiveness; there are no examples of Jesus withholding relationship from anyone as a result of their illness.

Another example of faulty thinking that exacerbated participants' depressive episodes was provided by participants who spoke of their roots in 'a tradition that "Christians don't get depressed and you can't admit to being depressed and if you are, you can't have much faith if you're depressed...if you just love Jesus enough, you won't get depression." ' (Nora). Participants' internalization of these unfounded and unscriptural beliefs about Christianity subsequently tortured their self-esteem, their faith, and their understanding of God's love for them regardless of their illness.

The myth that 'Christians don't get depressed' undermined participants' identity as all were Christian *and* depressed. Both distant and close participants feared they would no longer be trusted with church roles and responsibilities once their weakness became public. Some participants desperately forced themselves to maintain a good outward visage to prove that they were 'good enough'. This striving resulted in further fuelling of participants' depression. Losing valued roles and responsibilities would further undermine their identity and compound the loss of meaning and self-worth inherent in depression. The theological challenge in this context would be to the reference of God's unconditional love for His creation (Ephesians 3:18–19).

Many participants referred to the need for a reason to be depressed. This may reflect a personal struggle to accept the temporarily altered change of identity and behaviour that accompanies depression. If so, this is a challenge to the second great commandment: to love ourselves as we love each other (Matthew 19:19). Depression is replete with challenges to one's faith; how these challenges are resolved by an individual will reflect inwardly on the person's relationship with God (Fowler 1981, 2004) and reflect outwardly as faith being a hindrance or a help during an episode of depression (Pargament and Ano 2004).

The above discussion suggests that negative effects of faith on depression may be products of individual thinking patterns learned through various life situations. Learned thinking patterns and belief systems prevail in the first instance during life's difficult times, such as when depression occurs and when the person's world and life are seen to 'fall apart' (Beck 1967). Negative thinking patterns are individualistic and are not accepted Christian beliefs or biblical teachings. Although at times faith is held responsible for exacerbating depression, it can be argued from the most basic theological viewpoint that these claims are not founded in accepted biblical teaching.

Participants of both close and distant groups discussed decades of struggle with irrational ideas and faulty thinking patterns. Of those participants who received counselling, all from the close group and one from the distant group replaced negative thinking patterns and beliefs with a new understanding of God and the scriptures. Out of depression's 'pit of ashes', this new revelation of God's nature provided participants with a new positive perspective on life which gave them 'joy' that had not subsided.[3]

While distant-group participants knew the scriptures, all had formed an uncertain and hesitant concept of God's character and how this related to them as individuals; all expressed doubts about God's nature and therefore had not developed an applied trust in God for their daily lives. With lack of trust and therefore a distant relationship, these participants lacked a framework that enabled hope in a faithful God and hence found themselves at the mercy of the depressive episode.

Spiritual features of depression

Depression manifests through physical, emotional and cognitive expressions (Beck 1967; Kaplan and Sadock 1991) that collectively influence a person's spirituality (Paige 1994). While there are biblical examples of depression (Job, King David, Jacob), the scriptures suggest that God's choice for people's lives is 'plans for your welfare [good] and not for harm, to give you a future with hope' (Jeremiah 29:11), and 'I [Jesus] came that they may have life, and have it abundantly' (John 10:10b). However, John 10:10a provides the antagonist and one explanation of depression, 'The thief [devil] comes only to steal and kill and destroy'. Some common spiritual features of depression emerged through this study.

Also experienced and described by Paige (1994), a progressive deepening of physical and spiritual elements of depression was evident as the depressive spiritual influence settled over study participants. The following progressive stages were evident in participants' responses:

1. 'Somebody turned off the switch of my life': disconnection and alienation from God.

2. Is God deaf and mute? The one-way street, but which way?

3. 'Divided we fall, united we stand': self-isolation.

4. 'I feel I've let God down': guilty, twisted and unscriptural thinking.

5. 'I was angry with God and wrote Him nasty letters'.

6. 'Maybe I'm not a Christian after all': a cognitive triad.

7. Thoughts of self-harm.

'Somebody turned off the switch of my life': disconnection and alienation from God

A most distressing effect of depression on spirituality was a perception of separation from God, an abandonment that made participants feel as though they were in a 'Godless place'. Several participants described what might be considered a 'spiritual force' that overwhelmed them, severing their usual two-way spiritual relationship with God. Participants described this force in the following ways:

- Something comes over me, comes down on me.

- It's like a black cloud just covers me.

- It's like somebody turns off the switch of my life, and everything goes black.

- It's like a blockage.

- It's as though I'm sinking deeper and deeper into something black and I never know how far I will sink before it stops.

- It's like I'm a piece of dust, and I keep getting covered over more and more; I'm choking but I don't choke. I become transparent or something and people don't even know I am there.

Close-group participants in particular experienced severe distress as disconnection from God exacerbated their depression.

Is God deaf and mute? The one-way street, but which way?

Disconnection from God manifested as difficulty communicating with and hearing God's voice. Participants said that communication became either one-way or completely non-existent, but all agreed the problem was of their own making; they believed that God continued to make an effort to connect with them but they were unable to receive this or to reciprocate. As participants perceived an inability to communicate with God, they experienced increased difficulty praying and increased isolation from God. Participants felt they were carrying the burden of depression alone.

Participants who previously sensed God's presence through the scriptures found the blockage pervaded this potential source of connection with God. Depression affects concentration, so that reading is frequently incomprehensible (American Psychiatric Association 1994; Kaplan and Sadock 1991). This removed another potential avenue of connecting with God and deepened participants' sense of isolation.

'Divided we fall, united we stand': self-isolation

Approximately equal numbers from both groups self-isolated during depression, intentionally withdrawing from their supports, which made them more susceptible to deeper or longer depression (Evans, Burrows and Norman 2000). At least three of the female participants said they were glad their husbands were ill; 'it gave me an excuse to stay at home, and nobody knew the difference' (Helen). Under the influence of depression, participants felt socially 'unattractive' and preferred to avoid their church and social communities to preserve their acceptability. In retrospect, participants acknowledged the incongruence of self-isolation in their time of need.

Two participants described themselves as natural loners. As the depression worsened, loneliness assumed a painful bleakness. 'I know this would naturally make one seek company, but it doesn't.' This redoubling of their pain is a parallel experience to that of the participants who intentionally withdrew from social supports.

All participants who withdrew from potential social support retrospectively recognized how this action compounded their depressive episode, but at the time all were blinded to the potential support that others might bring. When not under the influence of depression, these participants reflected on the incongruence of their actions. This confusion adds credence to the suggestion that depression has a deep spiritual overshadowing.

The scriptures emphasize the importance of fellowship and relationship among the Body of Christ (Hebrews 10:25). Designed by a triune God as relational beings, we belong to a worldwide community to which we contribute and from which we garner support (Joyner 2005a, b, c). The connectedness of this community bears centuries of history and overcomes boundaries of nationality, economics and education. This deep sense of belonging can counter isolation and restore common goals for the depressed person (Gardner, Pickett and Brewer 2000; Joyner 2005a). 'Divided we fall, united we stand' is true from a scriptural perspective as well as a humanistic or secular perspective (Jackson 2006a).

'I feel I've let God down': guilty, twisted and unscriptural thinking

Some study participants said they felt responsible for disappointing God by being depressed and making it hard for God to help them, and consequently felt guilty for letting God down. This is well covered in earlier discussion regarding twisted and faulty thinking. Reflecting upon the unscriptural basis of their depressive beliefs participants recognized confusion and incongruence of thoughts and beliefs occurring during depression.

Scripturally, God's acceptance of us is neither earned nor susceptible to change (Ephesians 2:8–9; John 10:28–29).

'I was angry with God and wrote Him nasty letters'

Some participants revealed anger with God 'for letting this happen' and taking them out of their employment, routines, demeanour and familiar identities. Anger compounded participants' guilt and urged the need to self-isolate lest someone observed the participant's anger. This augmented the participant's self-perceived weakness as a Christian.

Other participants blamed themselves (whether genuinely or otherwise) thereby saving face for God. Theologically, God does not need our protection and condones appropriate expression of anger (Ephesians 4:26).[4] The confusion appearing earlier has been compounded to create a widening schism between the participant and God. Recalling the scripture of the thief coming to rob, depression emulates theft of participants' coveted relationship with God. Is depression the spiritual manifestation of 'the thief', or is it permitted of God, as was the suffering of Job or of Simon (Luke 22:31–32)[5]?

'Maybe I'm not a Christian after all': a cognitive triad

Depression caused many participants to question their faith or God's existence; their self-response confirmed participants' inadequacy as Christians and further exacerbated the depressive episode. This is an example of Beck's (1967) cognitive triad, a strategy by which the depressed person structures their perception of self and inevitable future. The triad consists of three partners: negative self-talk, twisted thinking and irrational (unfounded) thoughts or beliefs.

At this stage of deep depression, participants viewed their inability to connect with God as confirmation that God either did not exist or had turned

His back on them, or that perhaps they weren't a Christian at all. When not in depression, participants could see that the self-responses to their cognitive triad options were lies that brought them perilously close to self-destruction. For Paige (1994), 'the spiritual aspects are the most dangerous to our well-being. When we lose contact with God, we feel truly alone, and despair can become more inviting, death, more appealing' (p.41).

Thoughts of self-harm

Some participants 'prayed that God would take me in my sleep'. All participants believed that suicide was not an option but neither was the pain and suffering of continuing life in a Godless place, in the 'tunnel at the end of the light' (Paige 1994, p.20). Despair and hopelessness can culminate in self-harm (Clarke 2003; Hill *et al.* 1998) which is a potential outcome for those without hope in God (Touhy 2001). A known depressive illness is present in about 70 per cent of people who take their lives (Hickie *et al.* 2003).

Several participants discussed self-harm. About half of these took no action because of their faith in God while the others said they took strength from their families. Thoughts of self-harm are common in depression (American Psychiatric Association 1994; De Leo *et al.* 2001; Kaplan and Sadock 1991; National Institute of Mental Health Press Office 2005) and mirror the ultimate goal of 'the thief' who comes to kill and destroy.

Participants' experiences of depression clearly support an argument for depression having a spiritual overtone and certainly affecting the spiritual lives of Christians. This must draw a response from the church that has at least a pastoral role in nurturing a depressed congregant back into health. While not specifically focusing on older people, Swinton's study (2001) suggested that those depressed people who were nurtured through their depressive episodes by active Christians, recovered more quickly and maintained a healthier spiritual life through ongoing connectedness with the church. What then might be the response from the church?

Response from the church

Seventy-five per cent of participants said their church made some effort to help them during depression but 91 per cent of the close-group participants in this group said the church's efforts frequently resulted in more distress as those who came to help lacked understanding of the illness. While one participant valued the well-intentioned visit of her pastor and his wife, their questions and suggestions were unhelpful. 'I couldn't wait for them to go! ... so that time that I really needed the support, there were a couple of people who helped and there were a few that were absolutely no help at all' (Margaret). Assistance was frequently provided by a single person; at other times, the participant's home group nurtured the participant without involving the clergy.

All of the distant-group participants in this group said that they had felt unsupported by their churches. Of these, 66 per cent would not disclose their depression to their minister or other congregants through fear of shame and stigma and 20 per cent didn't attend church yet wondered why the church didn't respond to their depression in absentia.

While the 'unsupportive churches' claims of the distant participants proved unsubstantiated because these participants were not active attenders, the fact remains that close participants also felt their churches' responses lacked pertinence. If, through its prophetic abilities and discernment, a church perceived a congregant's depression and commenced appropriate action, would the church risk a slap in the face for being presumptuous, particularly since stigma and various fears are likely to have prevented congregant disclosure? The responsibility of the church in supporting a congregant through depression must be carefully considered and may vary among churches.

Having eliminated the suggestion that the church was *un*supportive, the issue clarifies to lack of appropriate church response through lack of understanding of depression and mental illness. One participant's words, 'I need someone to accept me and understand me, no matter what', suggest that the church culture might need review if congregants fear stigma and loss of acceptance through disclosure of a mental illness. Depression challenged the social expectation that Christians are happy people.

Half of the close group, and some of the distant group speaking on how the church helped them through depression, raised fears about disclosing their struggle with depression. A degree of non-disclosure was related to personal dignity and privacy but some participants feared rejection by the church family. The human need for acceptance and belonging (Meador 2004) was no different for this group of participants, many of whom said the church *was* their family, yet it was also where they were most afraid to be honest lest they 'lose their place' (Blazer, Sachs-Ericsson and Hybels 2005; Gardner *et al.* 2000; Jackson 2006b).

Another common misconception among participants was that depression was a psychotic illness that necessitated 'the green car coming round'. If participants who experience depression are proponents of such beliefs, might the church's lack of understanding of depression be much greater? Clearly depression remains an ill-understood and unacceptable illness within some churches.

'Coming alongside' older Christians during episodes of depression

While no participant specified the type of assistance and support they expected from their churches, several participants used words similar to 'someone to come alongside me'. This suggests that participants' needs during depression may be as simple as someone's presence with them; however, the 'someone' needs to understand depression and thereby know whether and how to respond or to be silent as required by the depressed person (Swinton 2001).

Table 13.1 shows suggestions offered by study participants as possible responses of a person coming alongside someone with depression. The table provides an evidential premise from which to develop bespoke companionship with someone in depression. It is important for the companion to remember that the episode of depression will pass, but is unpredictable with respect to severity or duration (Kaplan and Sadock 1991). Patience is essential.

Participants who forced themselves to attend church services while they were depressed said they valued fellow congregants who regarded them with the usual

Table 13.1 A starting point for coming alongside someone with depression

Difficulty	Possible response
Disruption of relationship and connectedness with God; feelings of alienation and abandonment	Become the conduit between the depressed person and God; just sit with them, **not necessarily talking**.
Difficulty communicating with God and hearing from God	Discuss how the person usually communicates with and hears from God. **Offer to pray with or for the person**, in the format with which they are familiar, or apart from them; allow the person to resume prayers as they are able. If words are difficult, then sighs or sounds may suffice (Romans 8:26), or spiritual music such as hymns may provide the spiritual expression required.

continued on next page

Table 13.1 continued

Difficulty	Possible response
Inability to read the scriptures	Read the scriptures, prayers or devotionals with and/or for the person. Remember concentration may be impaired, so think in **small doses**.
Isolation from church community and from others	Provide transport to and from church; be present for the person in church; visit the person in their home; find common ground on which to **connect**; resist giving advice, but **walk beside** the person.
Feelings of letting God down because they can't control the depression	Talk this through, referring to the scriptures or other sources familiar to the person; gently reaffirm God's nature towards the individual. Gently challenge unbiblical beliefs.
Anger with God 'for letting this happen'	Accept the expression of anger as healthy and biblical (Ephesians 4:26). **Accept the person** regardless of silence or emotion. Encourage the person to talk as they are able.
Questioning of their faith; negative thinking – worthlessness, hopelessness, poor self-concept, self-blame, guilt etc.	Help the person find positive exceptions to their examples to encourage them and provide hope. Listen without condemnation, but with **honesty. Provide hope and a safe environment to talk**.
Internal dilemma between struggling to fight the depression versus letting go, trusting God	Listen; be present for the person; encourage them through the scriptures; confirm the loving and compassionate nature of God.

level of respect. Related to the depression, these participants were frequently fragile and emotional over long periods of time and sought the congregation's acceptance without undue fuss over the participant's emotional state.

Whether individually or corporately within a congregation, the most important thing is to connect with the depressed individual without intruding into their personal life; to accept them unconditionally and continue to include them in usual activities. Participants said they did not need to be controlled or advised; they were already acutely aware of having lost control and were trying to maintain a semblance of 'normal' life regardless of depression.

The end of the line

Talk of self-harm or suicide is an inner expression of deepest emotional pain for which the person cannot find an alternate expression or solution. Assisting someone to talk about suicide is healthier and safer than suppressing that discussion and will not motivate action.[6] Enabling people to release their pain is the first stage of abating the person's inner turmoil[7] as such discussion alleviates potential avenues of guilt.

It is common for the listener to feel overwhelmed or uncomfortable with talking about self-harm, in which case help can be sought from professionals or from a range of current websites, some of which are listed at the end of this chapter.

Conclusion

This chapter presents some findings of a recent qualitative study that explored the interplay of depression and Christian faith in the later life of 20 Christian participants. The study group showed a high level of homogeneity for depression, but varying degrees of relationship with God. Participants with a closer relationship with God had progressed further in their faith development and while their episodes of depression were possibly worse than distant participants, close participants found comfort and strength through practical application of their faith. This was only possible for those participants who were able to trust God as a close friend.

The most devastating effects of depression on faith resulted from a perceived severance from God and subsequent feelings of increased hopelessness accompanying a growing sense of abandonment. During depression, participants acted in ways contrary to usual behaviour when not depressed. These behaviours exacerbated the depression and attested to a spiritual influence with a goal of separating the participant from God, and in some instances, from the support of their churches. Spiritual features of depression were discussed within a theological context.

Participants with a close relationship with God found that their church's response to depression was inadequate and participants from the distant group reported no support from their church. Although this claim proved unfounded, the majority of study participants perceived their churches as unsafe environments in which to disclose depression; stigma and lack of acceptance were feared by many participants.

The overarching need expressed by participants was unconditional acceptance and respect as if they were not depressed. This chapter has presented initial approaches to someone experiencing an episode of depression, enabling the revelation of God amidst the pit of ashes. From those who have been there and back through depression, this God is personified in someone who is able to connect, not give advice, but walk beside; not intruding; rejoicing with me and crying with me; listening to me, not condemning me; someone who talks to me honestly; someone who doesn't offer advice, but just sits with me; encourages me; is present with me; accepts me however I am … It's 'Jesus in a skin'.

While this chapter has provided some initial suggestions for immediate contact with a depressed person, the reader may be drawn to consider training in pastoral counselling, or programmes that might enlighten the understanding of various mental illnesses. Basic suicide awareness training might also be advantageous.

Website references for suicide prevention and education

American Foundation for Suicide Prevention: www.afsp.org

Australian Institute for Suicide Research and Prevention (AISRAP):
    www.griffith.edu.au/school/psy/aisrap

beyondBlue (Australian National Depression Initiative): www.beyondblue.org.au

ybblue (the youth program of beyondblue): www.beyondblue.org.au/ybblue

Centre for Suicide Research (University of Oxford):
    http://cebmh.warne.ox.ac.uk/csr

International Association for Suicide Prevention (IASP): www.med.uio.no/iasp

Mind (UK): www.mind.org.uk

National Institute of Mental Health (USA): www.nimh.nih.gov

World Health Organization (WHO): www.who.int/mental_health/en

WHO Suicide Prevention and Special Programs:
    www.who.int/mental_health/prevention/en

Notes

1 'We know that all things work together for good for those who love God, who are called according to his purpose': Romans 8:28, New Revised Standard Version, 1989.

2 At www.quotegarden.com/teen-heart.html.

3 'To provide for those who mourn in Zion – to give them a garland instead of ashes, the oil of gladness instead of mourning, the mantle of praise instead of a faint spirit': Isaiah 61:3, New Revised Standard Version, 1989.

4 'Be angry but do not sin; do not let the sun go down on your anger': New Revised Standard Version, 1989.

5 'Simon, Simon, listen! Satan has demanded to sift all of you like wheat, but I have prayed for you that your own faith may not fail; and you, when once you have turned back, strengthen your brothers': New Revised Standard Version, 1989.

6 See www.betterhealth.vic.gov.au/bhcv2/bhcarticles.nsf/pages/Suicide_and_mental_illness_explained.

7 Australian Institute for Suicide Research and Prevention, Suicide Prevention Skills Training Workshop, www.gu.edu.au/ school/psy/aisrap/.

CHAPTER 14

Hearing the Voice of the Elderly: The Potential for Choir Work to Reduce Depression and Meet Spiritual Needs

Kirstin Robertson-Gillam

Introduction

A pilot study was carried out to test the potential for choir work to reduce depression and increase quality of life in elderly people with dementia, living in residential care, and to analyse the extent to which it met their spiritual needs.

The participants in the study were randomly assigned to three groups: the choir group; the reminiscence group, to test choir work against an established therapy; and the waiting list group, who continued to receive the normal facility care and who were used as a comparison against the other two groups. At the end of the study the waiting list group was given the choice of joining one of the other two groups. The choir and reminiscence groups met once per week for 20 weeks.

Participants were assessed for depression using the Cornell Scale for Depression in Dementia (Alexopoulos *et al.* 1988), for cognitive mental states using the Mini Mental State Examination (MMSE) (Folstein, Folstein and McHugh 1975), and for quality of life using the Alzheimer's Disease-Related Quality of Life Index (Rabins *et al.* 1999) before, during and after the study.

Forty-five participants, with an average age of 80 years, from The Hammond Care Group's aged care facility in southwestern Sydney, Australia, consented to participate in the study. Two-thirds of the participants had a diagnosis of dementia while one third-did not.

Illnesses, deaths and movements between groups resulted in a final sample of 29 participants across the three groups with 18 females and 11 males. The small sample size made the achievement of statistically significant results difficult. However, there was a positive trend towards reduction of depression and improvement in quality of life. This led to plans for the replication of the study as a controlled trial with university ethical consent, using a dementia-specific population.

Qualitative results indicated increased levels of motivation and engagement. Learning increased as the song lyrics evoked long-term memories with religious and spiritual meanings for many choir members. The reminiscence group gave participants the opportunity to revisit and resolve earlier conflicts in their lives through interactive group conversations and creativity.

Depression: a major problem in aged care?

Fleming (2004) found that 51 per cent of residents in high-care homes for the elderly demonstrated symptoms of depression as measured by the Geriatric Depression Scale (Yesavage *et al.* 1983). Furthermore, Llewellyn-Jones (2004) stated that depression in later life is a 'public health problem' affecting up to one in five elderly residents.

Depression is the most frequently occurring emotional disorder in older adults. A major depressive disorder in the old age range is found in 2–10 per cent of that population (Blazer, Hughes and George 1987), while 20–30 per cent of older adults were found to suffer from milder depressive symptoms (Butler, Lewis and Sunderland 1991).

Anderson (2002) noted that the general belief of depression being a normal part of growing old is 'categorically flawed' as well as being 'unethical', even though depression is closely associated with the ageing process. Many old people have experienced a wide range of losses including bereavement, physically debilitating illnesses and decreased mental and physical energy. These factors put elderly people at risk of depression. Could depression be a precursor for dementia in older people? Kaszniak and Christenson (1994) noted that depression could be mistaken for dementia symptoms and therefore go undiagnosed.

Spirituality and religion

Knowledge and understanding of the deep spiritual and psychological processes that underlie our humanness are at the very root of creative activities with older people. Choir work can reflect a search for meaning that is spiritual in its essence (MacKinlay 2006b). When we find meaning and purpose, our personhood is validated.

All behaviour has meaning and is a form of communication. Participation in a choir can provide an opportunity for a person to succeed at learning a new skill. The task is offered in such a way that they can achieve at their own pace. Davis (2005) called this approach 'errorless learning', meaning that 'individuals are given tasks in which the likelihood of making mistakes is reduced, so that time and learning efforts are not wasted by reinforcing incorrect information' (p.305). This approach can 'help individuals maintain their quality of life as long as possible' (p.304).

This social learning idea is important in choir work, where learning to sing correctly can become a source of anxiety from earlier conditioning. Bird and Luszcz (1993) used categorical cues to help memory recall and found that 'the same information presented as a cue both at encoding and recall' facilitates 'self-cues for memory and performance' (p.307). In choir work, elderly people with and without dementia can follow verbal cues and specific actions as modelling for remembering tasks. This approach reduces any anxiety associated with learning a new skill and provides enjoyment in the process of mastering it.

Research indicates that people who enter residential care are encouraged to embrace the 'patient-as-victim' role that can lead to learned helplessness and mental illness (Sperry 1992, p.398). Choir work encourages elderly people to give back to their community by performing at special events. This is in contrast to the regular practice of being entertained by younger artists. Even though there is great benefit in having such entertainment presented to elderly residents, it can be balanced by their own contributions adding more meaning and purpose to their lives. Singing hymns in a choir performance at special events such as Easter and Christmas can bring back past memories, foster spiritual expression and renew religious faith.

Similarly, reminiscence work validates an elderly person through giving the opportunity to explore their inner lives, relive their past memories and encourage time for reflection. This process fosters spiritual expression.

Aspects underlying choir work

Spirituality

Spirituality defines the uniqueness of people and draws out their innate creative abilities. It is now well known that there is a connection between religious and spiritual health, influencing adaptation to life when faced with the stresses of old age (Isaiah, Parker and Murrow 1999; Koenig and Kuchibhatia 1999). Mauritzen (1988) observed that 'spirituality represents the dimension that contributes to the core of a person's being…the essence of one's self and existence' (p.234).

Kaut (2002, p.226) asserted that 'the very act of remembering and recollecting the important and meaningful events of one's life, allows an entrance into the spiritual'. Spirituality can involve a personal quest for seeking understandings about major existential questions such as 'Who am I?', 'What is my purpose in life?' or 'How do I fit into the world?' (Frey, Daaleman and Peyton 2005, p.559). At some stage of our lives, we seek to transcend the 'ordinary' of everyday existence and yearn for the spiritual.

In choir and reminiscence work, the emphasis is on developing the untapped creative potential in elderly people, with a focus on 'positive subjective experience and depicting spirituality as providing a framework for adjustment, growth, and reaching one's human potential' (Snyder and Lopez 2002, p.559).

Religion

Koenig, McCullough and Larson (2001, p.18) asserted that religion is an organized system of beliefs, practices, rituals and symbols that help people to transcend the ordinary and believe in a greater power. Religious organizations foster social and community relationships as well as helping the individual to come to terms with their relationship to themselves and their God, whatever that concept may mean at a personal level. There are many different religions in the world. We need to understand the cultural and social significance of each religion and its origins, in order to learn tolerance and understanding between different cultures.

Religion and spirituality are interconnected. They point towards the transcendent qualities of existence, speaking about the sacredness of life or the beauty of nature. Spirituality can be seen as a search for meaning through relationships, nature and the arts – such as music, art and dance (MacKinlay 2006a, p.126). There is a growing awareness of the universality of spirituality and its formal expression in religious practices, both of which help to define meaning and purpose for human beings.

Creativity

'Creativity belongs to being alive' (Winnicott 1986, p.41). This refers to meaning, purpose and the drive for psychic wholeness. It can represent a way to address and resolve dissatisfactions in life. According to Winnicott (1986, p.51), 'experience can be creative and can be felt to be exciting in the sense that there is always something new and unexpected in the air'. This describes the atmosphere at the Hammond Village every Monday morning as people arrive in the chapel for choir practice. One choir member continuously says that 'choir is my medicine'.

Creativity in later life optimizes a person's functioning in the face of growing disease and disability (Nakamura and Csikszentmihalyi 2003). Old age, for some, can represent physical, cognitive, social and emotional constraints, all of which have the potential to strip a person of their creative nature and their essential personhood. Participating in a choir can enable an elderly person to be creative through the sheer enjoyment of singing with others and discussing life's memories evoked by the song material.

Inside each one of us is a spark similar to the flame of a candle. This is our essence: the spiritual aspect of our personhood (Killick 2006). Killick quoted this idea from a poem by a woman with early dementia, Barb Noon (in Killick 2006, p.75; see also p.126 in this volume), in which she expressed how she loses a little bit of herself every day, as the candle becomes smaller but the flame keeps burning just as brightly. Throughout our lives, the flame burns brightly whether we are living to our optimum potential, or during illness and trauma, or at the end of life.

Creative approaches are able to make the flame more visible and present, thereby broadening horizons for people who thought that they could no longer contribute to life. Through creative activities, elderly people can find meaning and purpose once more.

Imagination

There is the potential to have a rich inner life filled with imagination and creative thought across the lifespan. It has been suggested by Perlmutter (1988) that the psychological traits which are connected to creativity and which involve imagination remain in the consciousness until late in life. Creative activities such as singing, music-making, telling stories, writing and reading poetry, having tea parties, doing scrapbooking and handling soft toys are all used as conversational objects. They provide avenues for stimulating the imagination and creative abilities of people with dementia and disabilities, as well as helping them to find personal meaning and purpose.

Creativity expresses the transcendent, spiritual dimension of people and serves as a reminder of such important aspects of what it is to be human: spontaneity, laughter, joy and self-expression.

Methodology of pilot project

Consents were obtained from the participants and their families or guardians. The consent process and ethical considerations were monitored by the management of The Hammond Care Group.

Baseline assessments were carried out and the participants were randomly assigned to one of three groups: choir, reminiscence or waiting list. The assessments involved testing for symptoms of depression and quality of life using the Cornell Scale for Depression in Dementia (Alexopoulos *et al.* 1988) and the Alzheimer's Disease-Related Quality of Life Index (Rabins *et al.* 1999) as well as for levels of cognitive functioning using the MMSE (Folstein *et al.* 1975). All participants were interviewed by the researcher before the interventions commenced, using a modified form of the Spirituality Index of Well-Being (Daaleman and Frey 2004).

Each group originally contained 15 people but illness, deaths and movements between groups, resulted in a final sample of

- choir – 12

- reminiscence – 10

- waiting list – 7.

There were 18 female and 11 male participants with a mean age of 80 years. Two-thirds of the participants had a diagnosis of dementia.

The participants were drawn from six different residential areas of the Hammond Village including

- two main nursing homes

- two dementia-specific hostel complexes

- palliative care nursing home

- self-care units

- main non-dementia hostel.

The interventions occurred weekly for 20 weeks. The reminiscence group was divided into two to allow for more conversational intimacy. Each session was evaluated by an additional assessment instrument developed by the researcher, the Music Therapy Quality Of Life Evaluation Form, containing items concerned with quality of life and recording participant comments with a Likert scale.

Mid-project assessments were carried out after ten weeks of interventions using the Cornell Depression Scale for Dementia and the Alzheimer's Disease-Related Quality of Life Index.

Post-assessments were done using the same instruments as well as the modified Spirituality Index of Well-Being as an interview tool.

Aspects of choir work

Techniques involved in choir work included relaxation with breath awareness, vocal improvisation, singing exercises and group singing. These techniques help to provide a change of perception, in which elderly people are helped to shift their focus from helplessness and depression, to motivation, learning and creative achievement.

For those who like to sing and discuss life's memories, being in the company of like-minded people can improve their awareness of personhood which may have diminished due to a dementing or other age-related condition. One choir member with late stage dementia told me that 'I have to sing in order to be understood'.

Learning a new skill

Choir work involves learning a new skill. It seems that human beings always rise to new challenges, no matter how young or old they may be. When an elderly person is enabled to find 'their voice' again and realize that they can still achieve, they are more likely to re-engage in life with increased meaning and purpose. Their depression may be lifted as a result.

The desire to sing and be part of a group are the main criteria for joining the choir. Learning *how* to sing comes next. Becoming silent and listening to the breath provides a contrast to the singing. It helps choir members become focused and is a welcome relief to the continuous noise factor that often pervades an aged care facility. Singing exercises strengthen throat and lung muscles and enable expansion of the vocal range.

Relaxation and breath awareness

McBee (2003) used mindfulness meditation with groups of frail elderly residents and found that they experienced solace and spiritual support through the practice of breath awareness. This type of meditation is practised in silence. Similarly, choir practice always begins with a few moments of silence, followed by deep breathing exercises to loosen up throat, chest and shoulder muscles. All choir members take part and the silence that ensues is meaningfully deafening! This part of choir work helps to reinforce personhood by giving time for reflection and contemplation. It also reduces stress and enhances singing.

Singing exercises and vocal improvisation

Austin (2001) observed that vocal improvisation could help to facilitate spontaneity and emotional expression. Singing exercises explored the length and breadth of the voice and allowed room for creating spontaneous vocal sounds. Many choir members became more interactive and communicative with each other as a result, and were more spontaneous about expressing their emotions.

The singing exercises provided a 'consistent and stable musical environment that facilitates spontaneity and emotional connection to self and others' (Austin 2001, p.144). Clair (2000) observed that elderly people tend to express dissatisfaction with their vocal quality, presumably due to the ageing process. However, over time, the vocal quality of the choir improved and the elderly voices have begun to sound pure, clear and young.

The song material

The song material was carefully chosen from the cultural, social, religious and spiritual aspects of the community in which the elderly people live. Some songs in the repertoire were not familiar to all choir members but they all showed surprising willingness to learn these songs.

The choir in this pilot study was predominantly Anglo-Celtic Christian, an aspect which influenced the choice of songs. A wide range of songs was offered from the spiritual, religious, jazz, classical and popular genres. They were presented in keys that were compatible with the elderly voice range. This ensured that the choir members were more able to sing in tune and reinforced Davis's (2005) idea of 'errorless learning' in which 'the likelihood of making mistakes is reduced' (p.305).

Singing involves language and music. It is a 'dynamic event that requires an interaction of a text with rhythmic and melodic motion of tunes' (Johnson and Ulatowska 1996, p.155). Song lyrics are poems set to music, involving the complex processes of cognition and abstraction along with the desire for beauty and spiritual expression.

People with dementia in the choir were able to attend and focus for one hour each week without becoming disturbed or restless, provided they were constantly supported and prompted. This could possibly be attributed to the enjoyable nature of singing coupled with how it touches the human spirit. Winnicott (1971, p.13) wrote that 'no human being is free from the strain of relating inner and outer reality, and that relief from this strain is provided by an intermediate area of experience which is not challenged, such as the arts or religion'. Perhaps the complex process involved in the act of singing could encourage the elderly person to rediscover 'the self' once more. As Winnicott (1971, p.54) stated, 'it is only in being creative that the individual discovers the self'.

Song lyrics tell stories about life, relationships, feelings and many other issues that people are reluctant or unable to speak about (Robertson-Gillam 1995). Many choir members with dementia can remember and sing the lyrics with fairly high levels of accuracy. This phenomenon is supported by Peretz *et al.* (2004) who quoted Halpern's (1988, 1989) observations that non-musicians are found to be highly consistent in their ability to sing familiar songs and that they exhibit precise memory for both pitch and tempo.

Before the pilot project commenced, song books were compiled and copyright permissions were obtained. This was a lengthy and arduous process. The music was also presented on the adjoining page to the words for those who could read music and follow the melody line. It was surprising how many choir members with dementia could still follow and read the words correctly. Some participants with severe dementia who had lost their reading ability showed great initiative in lip reading and following the conductor's instructions. This enabled them to sing most of the words correctly with prompting.

Performance events

Choir singing is about performance and needs an audience. Choir practice occurred once per week in the Village chapel for one hour during the pilot study. Since the pilot study, the choir has continued to improve and has given regular performances in front of residents, relatives and carers.

The Hammond Village Choir has been going for fourteen months at the time of writing and has performed at events including World Prayer Day, Easter, Christmas in July, Gospel and Jazz concerts, and Christmas Lessons and Carols Service.

They also performed for the Aged Care TV Channel Program, and a journalist from a major Sydney newspaper wrote an article entitled 'Songs to Remember' (Scobie 2006). Media interest in the choir also added to purpose and meaning for the members. They felt that they were no longer isolated and forgotten but were continuing to participate meaningfully in their society.

Two choir members

Jim[1] suffered from Parkinson's disease and could not swallow. He was losing his power of speech and suffered from depression and isolation, but not dementia. Jim joined the choir so that he could begin to use his throat muscles again in the hope that this would improve his ability to verbally communicate.

After 12 months in the choir, Jim's speech improved enormously and his self-esteem and confidence increased. His loved ones and carers were amazed at the difference. Jim began attending individual vocal therapy as well as choir and this improved his communication abilities even more. He did not suffer from depression as much and felt that he had something meaningful to do in his life. The choir gave him a real purpose, especially during performances at special events such as Christmas and Easter services and other celebrations. Jim felt that he was giving back to his community and had more control over his life.

Arthur[1] was a very strong and physically fit man with severe dementia and challenging behaviours. He lived in a dementia-specific hostel. He joined the choir because his wife and staff thought it might help his agitation. His wife said he loved music.

Arthur formed a meaningful relationship with me in my role as choir leader. When he displayed signs of challenging behaviours during choir practice, such as shaking his leg, rustling his papers and becoming angry, I was able to immediately intervene creatively with clear prompts, positive reinforcements, direct eye contact, and conducting the singing. This approach helped Arthur to enjoy moments of creative, spiritual ex-pression that enhanced his life.

Life review reminiscence

The reminiscence group of 10 was divided into two smaller groups to allow for more intimacy and conversation. There was a similar distribution of one-third of people without dementia to two-thirds with dementia as in the choir. However, in the second ten weeks of the study, this was reviewed due to the reluctance of some participants without dementia to attend. The two groups were then designated non-dementia and dementia-specific respectively. This was found to be more workable and still continues at the time of writing.

Putting one's life in order is central to the life review/reminiscence approach outlined by Gibson (1998). It relates to unresolved business that may end in late life despair (Erikson, Erikson and Kivnick 1986). The life review reminiscence group included creativity as well as storytelling and sharing.

Aspects of life review reminiscence

The tea party

Matching crockery of English rose design was used along with tablecloths and attractive afternoon tea food. Elderly people respond well to the tea ritual because of its familiarity with earlier memories of such social events. This helped to relax participants and encourage conversation.

Objects for stimulating conversation and learning new information

The idea of using objects to stimulate conversation has been found to work well with people who have dementia and feel lost and confused. It also is successful with elderly people who do not have dementia because it stimulates conversations, expanding their topics of interest.

Conversational objects can be many and varied. Examples include sea shells, the latest news events, stories, poems, driftwood, photos, drawings, scrapbooks, dolls, toy animals, and so on. These objects provide symbols that represent real life events and enable participants to express their ideas, feelings and existing knowledge with others, sharing as a group and deepening their inner thinking processes. For instance, the life and habits of animals evoked many lively discussions and provided a centrepiece for feelings of security, familiarity and conversation.

Life stories – about learning new information in reminiscence work

Mavis[1] was 100 years old, quite deaf but cognitively aware. She did not have dementia. She came to the reminiscence group every week and brought her travel journals. She shared her life story through the pages of her journals and was supported by the group when her deep grief and loss issues arose.

She also became very animated when asking for new information. One day, we were talking about the behaviour of sea creatures, particularly fish. The conversation became focused on the mating behaviour of whales. 'How do they make love?' she asked. 'It must be a sight. They're so big.' This topic caused quite a stir in her hostel as I gathered information about the mating behaviour of whales over a few weeks, and much laughter ensued.

Mavis was able to review her life and resolve much unfinished business as she attended reminiscence each week. She was counting the weeks to her 100-and-six-months-old milestone. At this time, she was asked by a TV reporter from the Australian Aged Care TV Channel about the secrets of living a long life. She said: 'Go out and enjoy your essence in the beautiful world. Live and enjoy your life. Bed is for sleeping at night. Sleeping during the day is baloney.' After the interview she told me that she didn't want to live to be 101 years old. She died suddenly but peacefully two days later. A wonderful closure for a long and interesting life.

Humour in reminiscence work

Conversations in reminiscence with people who have dementia can be stimulated by the use of humour in relation to conversational objects.

Doris[1] was examining a toy New Zealand sheep with a black face and dark eyes while the tea was being served. I engaged her in conversation about the sheep. She said 'But its eyes are hidden.' I replied that I didn't think this meant that New Zealand sheep couldn't see. She replied 'Perhaps they need glasses.' We had a hilarious moment when a staff member put her glasses on the sheep and everyone considered this possibility. I then suggested that perhaps sheep didn't need glasses because they didn't get short-sighted. She replied 'How do you know they don't get short-sighted? We don't know, do we!' I suggested that perhaps we might be able to tell if they bumped into fences or stumbled in the field. We all laughed at this possibility. Three months later, Doris repeated this idea as her own when she was once more engaged with the sheep. This suggested that some long-term memory pattern had been stimulated, perhaps because of the humour that had surrounded the original situation.

Assessments and results

The Mini Mental State Examination

The Mini Mental State Examination (Folstein *et al.* 1975) showed a moderate level of dementia across all three groups of the final sample of 29 participants, i.e., 17 out of a total score of 30.

The Cornell Scale for Depression in Dementia

The Cornell Scale for Depression in Dementia (Alexopoulos *et al.* 1988) was used with all participants before, during and after the interventions. All groups showed scores below the indication for symptoms of depression at baseline (see Figure 14.1). In order for symptoms of depression to be recognized, a score of over eight must be shown.

The choir group's scores increased at mid-project and then decreased at the end of the study, indicating that depressive symptoms increased before they decreased as a result of the intervention. One theory could be that the mid-assessments were carried out after Christmas when there was a break. It is possible that post-Christmas events could be responsible for causing a decrease in mood.

Another theory could be that the choir faced the challenges of learning a new skill while the other groups did not. Perhaps learning a new skill in the initial period could produce depressive symptoms as part of the learning process? This question was not answered by the pilot project. The reminiscence scores were lowest post-study while the waiting list group remained the same,

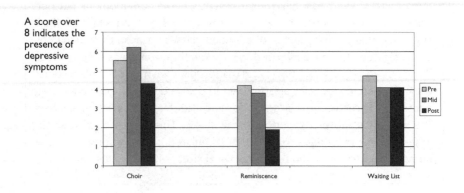

Figure 14.1 Cornell depression scores at the beginning, middle and end of the study, showing decreasing levels of depression in the choir and reminiscence groups only

indicating no change. Old people like to talk about themselves and their lives. Reminiscence is well known to be effective in this way (Gibson 1998).

The ADRQL

The Alzheimer's Disease-Related Quality of Life Index (Rabins *et al.* 1999) was also used before, during and after the interventions. There were slightly higher scores for the reminiscence group post-study. Both choir and reminiscence scores increased while the waiting list scores decreased (see Figure 14.2). However, all changes in scores were very small so that no definite conclusion could be drawn from them – except that a positive trend was noted towards increasing quality of life.

The Spirituality Index of Well-Being

The Spirituality Index of Well-Being (Daaleman and Frey 2004) is a valid and reliable 12-item instrument that measures 'a dimension of spirituality linked to subjective well-being in patient populations' (Frey *et al.* 2005, p.558). It was originally developed in 2004 with an aged care population using qualitative research methods (Frey, Daaleman and Peyton 2005). It has six items which focus on self-efficacy and another six which focus on life schema. A modified version of the Likert scale was used to accommodate the needs of elderly people living with disabilities, including dementia.

The scores showed that the choir group had a slightly higher level of purpose than the other two groups (see Figure 14.3).

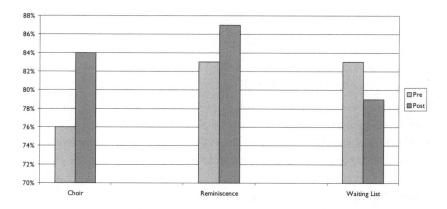

Figure 14.2 Alzheimer's Disease-Related Quality of Life Index scores at the beginning and end of the study, showing small increases in quality of life for the choir and reminiscence groups only

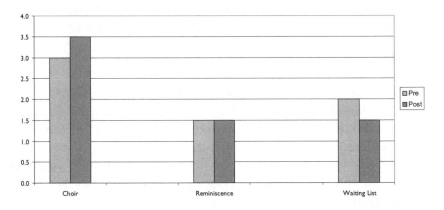

Figure 14.3 Spirituality Index of Well-Being scores at the beginning and end of the study, indicating higher levels of purpose and meaning in the choir group compared with the other groups

The following themes emerged from the participants' comments:

- grief and loss issues
- control over life situations
- predictions about imminent death
- past-time and 'real' present-time perspectives
- religious beliefs
- purpose and meaning
- family relationships
- work values
- values about the importance of education.

Levels of responsiveness to the active treatments

Responses to each session were videotaped and assessed using a Likert scale. Comments by participants and staff were also recorded. Quality of life aspects were itemized such as: levels of appropriate verbal and vocal communication during the singing or in conversations; motivation; self-esteem and self-confidence; expression of feelings; positive mood changes; social interaction; spontaneous helpfulness; and engagement levels during each session.

Measured responses were generally high across both groups. The choir group started below average and gradually climbed to high scores. This may have been due to the concentration required to learn a new skill and increased self-esteem as mastery became possible.

The reminiscence group indicated that awareness levels were consistent with exploring and processing past life experiences and events. The initial responses showed average scores but they quickly climbed to high scores and remained there. The waiting list was not included in these evaluations as they did not attend any of the interventions.

The results suggest that the effect of being part of a choir and/or reminiscence group was beneficial, with a positive trend towards reducing depression, increasing quality of life and spiritual meaning and purpose. There was an indication that with a larger sample size, statistically significant results may occur. Replication of the study is now being planned with a dementia-specific population in another facility owned by The Hammond Care Group.

Discussion

The project examined whether participation in a choir could reduce depression in elderly people with dementia in residential care, compared to a reminiscence group and a waiting list group.

Because there were small numbers, the statistical results were not significant, but there was a promising trend towards a decrease in depression and an increase in quality of life. The choir scores showed some interesting variations between baseline, mid- and post-scores that were not present in the reminiscence group. This may be due to the uniqueness of singing together and having a purpose to perform and take part in regular religious and non-religious events in the facility. Another explanation could be that singing may express the soul of a person and so is a deeply intimate and personal experience for many people. Being encouraged to sing may engender feelings of validation and self-confidence.

The main confounders in the pilot study were movement between groups, sicknesses and deaths which meant that 16 participants had to be deleted from the final sample, causing it to be too small to provide statistically significant results.

Scheduling session times for both groups had to fit in with various other activities such as hairdressing appointments, recreational activities and bus trips. All of this required considerable organization and coordination of six different areas of the Hammond Care facility. This also meant coordinating a large and diverse staff population, including primary care staff, pastoral care coordinators, educators, volunteers and music therapy students.

Elderly people in residential care have traditionally been expected to lead a passive and receptive lifestyle. However, the main aim of the choir and reminiscence groups was to help people find more meaning and purpose in their lives. This has been evident in the choir performances and camaraderie that ensued in both groups, during and after the study. Davis (2005) has suggested that 'education and behaviour interventions can be utilized to maximize quality of life as long as possible' (p.304).

Responses in the choir group showed a below average score at the beginning, with a gradual increase until most participants scored at the highest level near the end of the study. This indicated that learning occurred using verbal cues and modelling. Choir members demonstrated that they were able to remember tasks more easily as reported by their carers. This appeared to increase their motivation, self-esteem and confidence.

Comments by participants were collected and collated in response to 12 questions about self-perceived meaning and purpose in life. Some people in the choir commented on how singing helped to fill the emptiness in their lives and provide a better sense of self-efficacy and purpose. The reminiscence group's comments indicated elements of dealing with life's problems in constructive ways. The waiting list group's comments reflected some degree of depression and lack of meaning. This result correlated with Daaleman and Frey's assertion (2004) that 'provision of systems of meaning and coherence' could be associated with well-being and spirituality by participants.

In comparing the modified Spirituality Index of Well-Being results at the beginning and end of the study (see Figure 14.3), an observable trend towards the choir increasing the participants' well-being and sense of purpose was noted. The reminiscence group showed increased interest in learning new information and conversation, while the waiting list group showed some decrease in their quality of life.

Since the pilot project ceased, many people who were in the waiting list and reminiscence groups have joined the choir which now has a membership of between 25 and 30 people. Their performances are greatly enjoyed by the resident population and their families. The choir has now become an integral part of the life of The Hammond Village. A recent performance of Easter hymns and Bible readings evoked some tears of joy and meaning in some residents, while others were confident enough to sing some solo parts, much to the joy and appreciation of their families and carers.

Conclusion

The most encouraging result was the positive trend towards a decrease in depression with both choir and reminiscence groups. There was no change in the scores for the waiting list group. Further research is recommended with a larger sample in order to obtain statistically significant results. This research is currently being planned by The Hammond Care Group.

Choir work in aged care is challenging, deeply satisfying and very creative. It involves the spontaneous and the uninhibited, which exists within us all and expresses our timeless transcendent nature.

We all search for meaning, even in the face of severe hardship and suffering. Somehow, if we can find meaning, we can find life within the face of pain, discomfort, confusion and disability. We find God within us and come to realize that when we play and delight in the small precious moments of life, we are already there in the magical timelessness of forever. We become alive and live in that moment. It is only in each moment that we can live and have our being. Perhaps the elderly with conditions such as dementia and physical frailty have much to teach us about finding meaning in *being* rather than always *doing*. We become as little children and find our Christ-like natures within ourselves and each other. The world then becomes a playground of possibilities and discoveries until the day we die.

Note

All of the names used in the life stories have been changed to protect the identities of the people concerned.

CHAPTER 15

Humour and Its Link to Meaning and Spirituality in War

Carmen Moran

Introduction

Veterans of the Second World War are now in later life, and dealing with the common issues of ageing, including possible disability and deteriorating mental health. In this context they are also revisiting their experiences during the war, which may now be having an additional impact on them both physically and psychologically. This chapter looks at their war experiences, particularly the use of humour as discussed in reminiscences of their experiences, and the relationship of humour to past and current well-being. In this chapter I take the position that the use of humour serves different purposes at different stages of life, including extreme circumstances such as war. Humour can involve coping with here-and-now demands, but in later life it can become linked to a search for meaning. As a result, I suggest that humour may become more spiritually oriented in later life in the sense that it looks at meaning, rather than being distraction-oriented as it can be during times of extreme stress earlier in life.

The recollections and viewpoints from the interviews I present below are those of older people who were young adults during the Second World War. I do not deal to any extent with specific jokes or cartoons. Nor do I address the political aspects of war humour. While these aspects are part of the broad topic of humour and war, they are beyond the scope of this chapter, which is focused on the individual's experience of war and its effect on later life. I set humour in the context of stress and coping, and a search for meaning that encompasses war experiences from the perspective of older adulthood. This focus will, hopefully, be relevant to those who work with veterans, and perhaps those who work with older people in general.

People in later life have a range of experiences that they choose to review. In recent years, life review has been labelled 'autobiographical memory' or 'reminiscence' in the relevant literature (with the former term being more common in behavioural and memory literature, and the latter term more used in clinical or pastoral care literature). Reminiscence is often studied and applied in the context of theories such as Erikson's theory of psycho-social crises. Erikson's thesis is that each life stage presents us with a particular psycho-social crisis, and in later life that crisis is one of finding life's integrity versus despairing of life's meaning (Erikson 1963).

A large proportion of veterans of the Second World War were servicemen at an age associated with encoding memories that make up the period of the 'reminiscence bump'. During this period, approximately from adolescence to early adulthood, the person works on issues that ultimately make up 'the central components of an integral self', which are then most salient in later memory (Conway et al. 2005, p.740; Piolino et al. 2006). A tendency to focus on events of young adulthood in later life is common among all people, not just veterans. Nevertheless, veterans may have special needs in this regard given their 'integral self' was formed while serving in a war, and their reminiscences will reflect that.

As Coleman (1999, p.113) has noted, 'talking, thinking, and writing about the past can serve very different functions'. Humour can also serve different functions. In health-based literature there is a frequent assumption that humour always helps and is good for us, and that humour in the older person is a sign of good functioning. When that person is also a veteran of the Second World War, there may be a similar assumption that humour helped them cope during the war (Moran and Massam 2003). While such statements about the value of humour are accurate in part, they do not account for the different functions that humour can serve.

Challenging meaning is a characteristic of humour, and many writers see this as an important connection. Accordingly, the terms 'meaning' and 'spirituality' are being increasingly discussed in a range of articles. A search of the Internet using the terms 'humour and meaning' and 'humour and spirituality' reveals hundreds of thousands of articles. However, the same search on a scholarly database, such as PsycINFO, reveals fewer than thirty. This disparity shows that the widely promulgated claims about humour outweigh contemporary evidence and scholarship in quantity and also in quality. This does not mean carers and health workers should avoid humour in their work with older people while more research is done, just that a healthy level of critical appraisal is needed when it comes to popular assumptions about humour.

Veterans of the Second World War are now in their late 70s and early 80s, an age range associated with life review. For these men and women, dealing with and discussing their war experiences often comes after decades of personal silence. This silence contrasts with the stereotype of the garrulous veteran forever ready to discuss his past adventures. Those who work with veterans will recognize the former pattern as the more realistic, at least for most veterans. When it comes to formal discussions of humour and war, much more is written about veterans than is written by them. The interviews reported below were part of a project that sought to address that imbalance in respect to humour and its relationship to coping during war, including coping in later life. In this respect it is informed by a critical, but positive, perspective on mental health in extreme circumstances.

Humour may accompany, but not necessarily assuage, early stressful life experiences and the demands of later life. As health care workers will be aware, there is a growing literature on the persistence and late onset of post-traumatic symptoms in veterans of the Second World War (see below). Veterans are now at a stage of life where they are facing several growing challenges arising from normal aspects of ageing, as well as those related to disability, physical and psychological, brought on by war experiences. Any work on humour should not ignore this broad context in which veterans find themselves.

Definitions and theories of humour

Before looking further at the veterans, it may be worthwhile to outline what we mean by 'humour', especially for those who do not normally use humour in their work. There are numerous definitions of 'humour', varying from simple meanings, for example a stimulus, such as a joke, or a response, such as laughter, to more complex ones, such as cognitive processes involved in understanding and resolving an incongruity, or psychodynamic processes of accessing repressed pleasures. The different uses of the term make discussion on humour more complex than might appear at first. Furthermore, the numerous theories of humour are proposed from many scholarly perspectives, making the complexity even greater. On the other hand, humour is such a familiar concept that most of us think we understand what it is we are discussing. The need for clarity is more obvious in written rather than spoken discourse; clarity is also necessary for those wanting to articulate particular goals and outcomes when using humour in their work. In this chapter, humour most often refers to uses of humour *in situ*, such as witty remarks, jokes, or laughter. Hopefully the context will help clarify which aspect of humour is being discussed.

There are three sets of theories of humour that are relevant to this chapter, mostly because they help us understand that humour is not just about the laughter or internal processes. These theories also look at the way humour helps us deal with outside factors. In other words, both the internal and external aspects of humour are necessary to understand how people use and benefit from humour. For people working with reminiscence and life review, there may be other relevant theories among the many theories documented elsewhere (Ruch 1998).

The three sets of theories discussed here are the incongruity theories, the superiority theories, and the tension relief theories. The term 'sets of theories' is used because even within one type, for example the incongruity theories, there are various approaches to what is meant by incongruity and what its role is. Only a brief summary is provided; a fuller exposition can be found in Lefcourt (2001) and Martin (1998).

The incongruity theories tend to emphasize the way humour involves two scenarios that are normally considered incompatible. The humour arises because this incongruity is non-threatening, and the resolution, for example in a punchline, is pleasurable. When the incongruity is not resolved, there can still be pleasure when the combined scenario is seen as absurd.

The superiority theories emphasize the way in which humour allows us to feel superior to others, or to our former selves. Such humour may involve aggression. Some theories argue that humour always involves some element of aggression, but not all humour scholars would see humour this way. When humour does involve aggression, it is not always harmful, because such humour may help a person express feelings that could not readily be expressed overtly. Subversive humour, which is a form of aggressive humour, may even be a noble stand against a malicious leader or government.

Finally, the tension release (or relief) theories emphasize the way humour can lead to physical or psychological release. The physical release can come through laughter or other physical changes associated with humour. The psychological release can come through a cognitive process that involves altered perception, but this has yet to be fully explicated.

In the context of war, anything that assists the ability to deal with incongruity and absurdity, express aggression in a safe way, and help physical or psychological release would be valued by servicemen.

There is good empirical evidence that humour helps in dealing with current stress. The combined and separate work of Martin and Lefcourt, cited above, for example, has shown that various aspects of humour, especially 'sense of humour', are associated with lower distress in the face of stress. Such work has used humour questionnaires, as well as the ability to produce humour on demand. There is relatively little research on the long-term benefits of humour. Humour may be a lifetime coping strategy that represents a theme throughout life or humour may become more salient with a change of values as a result of life experience. These different aspects of humour will influence how the worker approaches the use of humour. For example, it may be difficult to draw out instances of humour from early adulthood in reminiscence work if the person was serious for the larger part of their lives. At the same time, experienced workers will be familiar with the fact that a current sense of humour often allows us to see something funny in the past that was not perceived as funny at the time.

Veterans, humour, and war

Several writers have looked at war-time humour. Mostly, they provide documentation on humour *about* war rather than humour *in* war (e.g., see articles in the collection of the Australian War Memorial, and Moran and Massam 2003). Such documentation is valuable, as it gives an insight into what people thought funny at the time, what they saw as fit to print, and what the focus of a nation was during those times. However, it would be too broad a leap to assume that the humour material that has survived today is the same as the humour used by servicemen in the fields of war, such as the desert or jungle, or in the camps. Even work seemingly done from the perspective of the serviceman often takes a broader political or sociological perspective, for example in Gerster's book *Big-Noting* (1987). This is not to say the effect on the serviceman is never considered, rather that the overarching framework is less about the individual and more about governments, organizations, or society in general.

In Australia some war documents, such as those archived in the Australian War Memorial and servicemen's private letters, have provided background material for understanding the personal use and appreciation of humour. More generally the public representations in books, films and songs inform the popular widespread view. This view asserts that sense of humour was inherent in the Australian soldier and frequently used, despite adversity and horror. Many still hold this view today.

There are, however, other views that challenge the popular view of humour in war. One perspective presents humour as part of the heroic mythologizing of the Australian soldier (as documented in Moran and Massam 2003). Anecdotes and tales of humour in war are seen as part of the propaganda associated with war, especially when the humorous tales are heroic, consolidating the notion of the fearless larrikin soldier. At the time, propaganda about servicemen's humour helped distance the Australian people from discontent and depression at the frontline. This propaganda was so effective that the image of the laughing soldier remained part of a national self-image, and even now is seldom challenged. The extent to which this stereotype impacts on veterans today as they attempt to look back at their war experiences remains generally ignored, and health care workers may find that veterans want to state their reality to contrast against the popular stereotype.

Humour among the servicemen was not always as innocent or cheerful as documented in official war books and magazines. For example, the humorous songs which were transmitted informally among servicemen often had explicit sexual references, profanity, and hostility. Popular public versions of the same song at home were much more restrained. There was also a range of tastes and levels of acceptance among servicemen. Veterans who went along with extremely sexual, sexist, racist and cruel humour may feel uncomfortable recalling this in formal reminiscence activities, especially in front of others who were 'not there'.

Coleman has noted how, in the relatively recent past, British health workers felt unable to deal with negative events or emotions experienced by older people giving their life story (Coleman 1999). In working with older veterans, experienced health care workers will be familiar with negative reactions and the need to challenge the stereotype of the laughing, easygoing soldier. This chapter seeks to assist both experienced and inexperienced workers with additional information from the veterans' perspective.

Research question

This chapter presents information collected as part of a larger study on humour, stress and coping in war. It addresses the specific research question 'How do Australian veterans of the Second World War view humour in war?' It was set in the context of a broader question 'How do veterans view those experiences today?' A further research question developed as this study occurred, namely 'How might any experiences of humour influence the current desire to revisit the broader aspect of war experiences and make meaning in the context of life review?' Although this study focused on Australian veterans, many of the readings and outcomes will have some relevance to soldiers of other nationalities or other wars, in the process of reviewing their life experiences (see Moran 2004).

Participants

The veterans in this study all participated voluntarily. They were men recruited from New South Wales (Australia) using a snowball technique. They had served in the following services: five from the Army (AIF, one POW), one Air Force (RAAF), and one Navy (RAN). They had experience of combat and being exposed to the dead and injured. The men's ages ranged from late 70s to mid 80s at the time of interview. The terms 'servicemen' and 'veterans' are used in this chapter for all services above. None was in residential care at the time, although that may have changed since the interviews.

The research was introduced to them as a study on humour in war, which was the original focus. Each participated in individual two-hour interviews. Margaret Massam did the interviews, and while initially directed at humour in war they were largely unstructured. The data below are incomplete due to her early death and the subsequent loss of full records and information about the participants. At first I put these data aside, because of their incompleteness, but I have decided that the outcomes from the interviews should be disseminated in recognition of the contributions and time the veterans were willing to give, and of Ms Massam's contribution. While conclusions must remain tentative as a result of the incomplete nature of the records for this study, there are some interesting issues that may help those working with veterans or others reviewing their lives.

Veterans' acknowledgment of humour

All participants acknowledged the presence of humour during their time as servicemen, including overseas at the front. Humour was variously regarded by them as a means of distraction, expressing feelings, subverting authority, bonding or 'mateship', acknowledging an enemy, providing physical release through laughter, or enjoyment for its own sake. This list is compatible with the various theories of humour, reinforcing the idea that humour does not serve one purpose, but can have various social, emotional and physical functions or consequences.

The veterans did not emphasize deliberate use of humour to alleviate stress. More often they spoke of another's humour that served this function. This pattern has also been noted in emergency work, where one person is often the wit or joker of the group and helps others laugh (Moran 2005). Hence, there is a need to distinguish between humour used to cope and humour which has the *effect of* enhancing coping.

An example of another's use of humour making servicemen laugh occurs in the following story told by one of the participants:

> After [a particular event]…the captain says '*Well, I got you out of that one*' and one person piped up '*You also got us into it*'.

Here, several men laughed and benefited from one person's ability and willingness to make a humorous comment in a time of stress.

Participants also discussed humour with reference to a situation where there was laughter rather than any special words that are recalled now. Many of the men spoke of someone falling into a latrine, and of the laughter this generated. It is not clear whether this is the one story that did the rounds, or it really did occur on several independent occasions. In contrast, similar stories of dysentery in the camps were told with sympathy.

The veterans all noted that there often was no place for humour. The idea that humour was ever-present, and the soldier could laugh in the most dire or stressful circumstances, was not supported in the interviews. Thus, humour may have served as a coping mechanism, providing social, emotional, and physical benefits, but as a coping mechanism it was limited in its effectiveness. Frankl (1984) highlighted the beneficial effect one person's humour could have on several other prisoners in the concentration camps of Nazi Germany. Importantly, however, he also stated that the beneficial effect of humour was transient. In other words, the effect of humour with camp prisoners was similar to that noted with our veterans.

The veterans' stories suggest that the effects of humour were limited across larger timeframes, as well as the shorter ones. That is, although participants reported it helped at the time, there was no sense that their war humour was of any particular benefit in any long-term way over the years. There was no mention of anyone resembling the Australian larrikin soldier laughing his way through war, emerging little changed psychologically. There were pleasant reminiscences about humour, but no belief that it prevented the subsequent effect of bad experiences.

Focus on war experience

All participants wanted to talk about past stressors or experiences, to the point that they changed the focus of the interviews away from humour. As a result, a larger proportion of the interviews were about the experiences of being servicemen and the stressors encountered. Not all stress was associated with combat, and frequent mention was made of uncomfortable conditions, poor health, and boredom. Some of the participants were still angry about the way they were treated. This anger was often towards the Service or officers, and related to equipment, planning and related facilities.

The participants recalled the sensations of 'being there' in the desert (dusty, hot, cold, remote) or jungle (wet, oppressive, unfamiliar). Their language indicated that the memories of negative aspects of the experiences were strong. However, these participants often mentioned that they had not talked about war since returning to civilian life many decades ago. They had only recently begun to talk, sometimes to let generations after them know what happened. In other cases, they did not explain why they were now talking about their war. In at least two cases this long-term silence about war experiences was verified by their wives. This pattern has been documented elsewhere in formal studies and is no doubt familiar to those who work with veterans on a regular basis (see below).

Why was there only a modest amount of humour discussed in interviews that had been presented as focusing on humour? We need to recall that much that is written about war humour is informed by, or contained in, fictional accounts in novels and films, or exaggerated accounts in propaganda or heroic mythologizing texts as discussed above. Recollections about humour in war can be found in other sources, and can include humour which is 'forced' (Johnston 2002, p.88) or part of a common parlance such as the 'slanguage' of soldiers (Laugesen 2003). Slanguage, or widespread use of special army slang, reveals less about war experiences than about the human tendency to play on words or speak in humorous jargon when members of special groups are together for a long time.

Humour in popular writing, especially newspaper accounts and novels sold to entertain, is often presented to the point of gross exaggeration. Moran and Massam (2003) cite examples such as Lambert's phrase 'terrible laughing men in slouch hats' and Laffin's assertion 'Women...emotions...rations...death... boredom – the standard Digger rule was to treat everything the same way; that is, laugh at it.' More moderate examples of humour written by servicemen themselves, such as George Sprod's (1981) *Bamboo Round My Shoulder: Changi, the Lighter Side*, remain the exception rather than the rule. The present interviews yielded accounts more like those in serious recent books rather than the popular views published at the time of the Second World War.

It is important, therefore, that we do not confuse the more numerous accounts *about* servicemen with accounts *by* servicemen, as noted earlier. In *At the Front Line*, Johnston (2002) has documented servicemen's discussions of their experiences in the Second World War. Humour gets only a minor mention among all their recollections. The few humorous items that are mentioned indicate abiding anger at the way they were treated at the time and after they were demobilized. In a similar vein, the servicemen-contributors to Barrett's book *We Were There* barely mentioned humour, and the term is not included in the index (Barrett 1995).

Then versus now

With any work relying on memory, we must recognize that the needs of the individual have changed and thus the nature and focus of recollections will have also changed. We need to recognize the needs of 'then versus now'. Thus perspective, not just memory alone, may explain different views of humour over time. In war (and its stressful aspects such as being far away from home, real or potential combat, risking life, extreme physical discomfort and so on) a type of humour is needed which provides an easy distraction or introduces a pleasurable event, even if only fleetingly. Humour may also serve other purposes, such as social bonding and emotional release. Regardless of type, it is reasonable to expect that a type of coping-humour was needed then. There was no evidence in the interviews that this type of humour was needed to any large degree now. This statement has to be qualified, because such a possibility was not directly canvassed in the study. We can say that the interview data indicate that talking about stressful war experiences, rather than humorous ones, is what is needed now.

Coping

Although the discussion on humour ended up being a minor part of these interviews, all participants agreed that humour occurred among servicemen. Even if the word 'coping' was not used explicitly, there was an understanding that humour helped them cope. Research on humour has shown that coping-humour has helped reduce distress across many stressful situations (Lefcourt 2001). It is possible that coping-humour can be too effective, for example in cases where humour has been associated with denial of disability or illness (Moran 2003). However, no relationship has been established here with servicemen's humour and any denial of their experiences.

Early coping does not necessarily predict later coping. Increasingly, health care workers, pastoral care workers, clinicians, and researchers are documenting cases of late onset post-traumatic stress disorder (PTSD) in veterans and survivors of traumatic experiences from the Second World War (e.g. Davison *et al.* 2006; Ruzich, Looi and Robertson 2005; Schnurr 1991). Labels other than PTSD may be used, but they commonly refer to severe symptoms linked to early-life events, such as war-related trauma.

On its own, a tendency to reminisce about war in later life does not indicate late onset PTSD. People who participated in the Second World War had experiences that constituted a major and dramatic focal point of their lives not only at the time, but many years later. For our participants, being a serviceman was associated with major changes in lifestyle, including extremely novel sights, sounds, smells, and other experiences, as well as exposure to possible or actual threats to well-being and to life. It is not surprising that these experiences would form a significant part of their life story in later life.

At the end of the war, servicemen embraced the national emphasis on a return to a normal life and most had a long period of stability. Admittedly, for some veterans such stability was more apparent than real, and others were unable to achieve even an appearance of stability. On balance, however, there was an emphasis on getting on with civilian life and the men went along with this. When reviewing their lives, freed from the emphasis on normalcy that occurred after the war, they now realize how profound and unusual that war experience was. From such a perspective it is not surprising that the veterans in our study now wanted us to appreciate their full war-time experiences, not just focus on humour.

Coleman (1999) has interpreted a similar pattern of a period of silence followed by a desire to talk in the following way: 'Silence occurred because war required a positive communal story, whereas later life reminiscence requires a personal story' (p.136). He reports that British veterans, and others such as civilians who experienced the London bombings, went along with the communal story for years after the war. The communal story was about stoicism and silence. Coleman focuses on people with disturbed mental health and disability, but the conclusions are similar to those in this chapter with its 'incidental' sample. He notes how personal stories were suppressed in the interest of appearing to cope, and this behaviour survived the post-war period. People only began to construct their individual life stories after retirement.

How people are heard may contribute to the benefits that result from now telling their stories. McKee *et al.* (2005) in their study of older people in residential homes found that reminiscence-based activities by care staff were not always associated with good health or well-being, and the outcome depended on factors such as unresolved regrets and how these were handled. The place of humour in reminiscence was not evaluated, but it may be that humour would have introduced a positive dimension to add balance to a focus on a negative aspect of people's lives. Furthermore, factors such as incongruity and tension release, which are properties of humour, can add to the flow of a story that may otherwise appear to lack structure or coherence. Humour, well managed by the care worker, may thus facilitate acceptance of a sort.

Distraction versus connectedness

While discussion of current humour was scant in our interviews, there was no evidence that our participants avoided using humour in later life. There are many different types of humour, and this study only canvassed personal humour related to war experiences. Appreciation of humour does not necessarily reduce with age and may even be more prominent (McFadden 2004; MacKinlay 2004). Differences have been found in specific humour-task-processing which reflects a cognitive decline (Shammi and Stuss 2003; Uekermann, Channon and Daum 2006). The latter types of studies use an artificial example of humour-processing within a laboratory context, and thus do not account for a broad range of humour in older people.

Depending on needs at a particular life stage or set of circumstances, the style of humour may change with age. At extremes suggested by this chapter, in the context of coping there may be two types of humour, labelled for our purposes here as 'blocking out' and 'integrating with'.

Psychologists and others have long speculated that humour can be used as a defence against others and against anxiety. This 'blocking-out' function explains humour's valuable function in war. This may not always be the case; for example, as one participant put it, 'Yes, we were scared at the time but laughed about it later'. More often, however, humour occurs at the same time as the stress, and laughter does not mean the stress is over. In war, and other extreme environments such as medical and emergency contexts, humour is described as a distraction. The terms 'blocking out' and 'distraction' are not pejorative because they refer to short-term effects that allow the person to continue with necessary and demanding activities. However, to outsiders the term 'distraction' can interfere with their understanding of how stressful a situation was; if a joke can easily distract people it must mean things are not that bad. People sometimes use that type of reasoning themselves – 'if I can laugh things can't be that bad'. In war, things can be that bad. In our sample, the veterans seemed to understand this perspective on humour. It did not give meaning to essentially meaningless or unavoidable negative experiences, but it helped them sustain a sense of value to their life. To them, humour at the time was more about blocking out, rather than filtering in, meaning.

Witty comments in the fields of war and gallows humour are examples of 'blocking-out' humour. As one interviewee commented,

> I can remember one funny incident [in a camp] when a train came through – it had a flat top and on the top were some Americans. We were very confused about what they were doing here but one called out 'Don't worry Aussie, Uncle Sam will be here soon.' Someone yelled back 'Don't tell me they've got him

too.' That produced a huge laugh. So despite being depressed, hungry, starving...

Humour can enhance interconnectedness with people. The social aspects of humour do not necessarily go beyond a passing sense of intimacy that can accompany shared laughter. In contrast, a deep sense of interconnectedness and life meaning occurs when humour has a certain type of message. Examples in contemporary work include certain Leunig cartoons, or jokes such as the following:

> A man is walking along the street in a distraught state. He prays 'God, please let me have $10, so I can buy some food and take it home to my family'. He looks up in supplication. He walks along a few metres, and finds a $10 note on the ground. He picks it up, looks up and says 'Don't worry God – I've found it by myself'.

At first glance this appears to be a joke about religion, but it is about meaning in a general sense. It uses the language of religion ('God', 'pray') but the humour comes from the mix of faith and hubris, the mix of an apparent trust in a divine and the lack of acceptance that divine intervention may actually have occurred. When we see this as the source of our laughter, the interconnectedness is with a spiritual self, rather than with other people, but we connect with others in our mutual recognition of our own tendency towards loss of trust and faith. There are other ways this joke could be interpreted, and that is the point about 'spiritual humour'. Such humour makes us look at life and its meaning, and the possibility of spiritual meaning. It is not about a correct interpretation of a joke (or cartoon etc.). Rather, it is about what we start thinking about as we appreciate the humour. The humour arises because of the structure of the joke, but the meaning comes from the specifics of the story within the joke.

Spiritual humour can occur in joking among friends, between health care worker and client, and so on. The nature of such informal interpersonal humour is often derived from non-verbal elements, and the words used in joking are seldom funny when written down. There may be a hidden message in joking, e.g. 'I care for you', 'I recognize you as a person', and so on, that does not come out in the words. In these instances, we use humour to integrate with our here-and-now experiences rather than block them out. Such humour occurred among servicemen too, but because of its ephemeral nature it was less readily documented than structured jokes. Because of its intimate nature, it may also be less readily shared with outsiders. In these interviews, the use of good-natured humour to help a fellow serviceman deal with something frightening or embarrassing showed this caring dimension in humour.

In the above examples, the *effect* of the humour becomes mixed with the *type* of humour, and it is not possible to separate these in any easy way. Examples of humour, whether blocking-out and integrating-with types, have to be accompanied by a fuller delineation of the person, the situation and so on, to explicate the type. There is a circularity set up whereby the humour is delineated in terms of its effect, which is presumed to arise from a type of humour. This problem of circularity becomes especially noticeable when discussing humour and meaning. It may be the sort of circularity that makes people working in health care despair of theorizing about humour, and to some extent they are correct. Practical, rather than theoretical, application of humour may help health care workers and their clients understand meaning in ways that are not readily articulated, yet still seen as valuable.

While the veterans of this study said humour helped them block out problems for a while, it is possible that humour also helped in other ways, including a more 'spiritual' way suggested here. That is, the humour helped them laugh with others, even when they were apparently laughing at others. There was a sense of 'we are all in this together'. This does not just lead to bonding, but also to compassion, an important quality in classical and contemporary views of spirituality.

A second question arises: Did humour help them find meaning in an often chaotic, incongruous, and demanding situation? Unfortunately, the interview data do not allow us to explore this possibility to any great extent. We can extrapolate from some of the veterans' statements, but more in terms of meaning derived after the war. For example, in the context of discussing humour one participant stated 'I think Australians can be very judgmental'. While this seems to be a criticism of fellow Australians, in context this statement showed how this veteran had moved to a stage where he judged others less, including soldiers who went AWOL, and the enemy.

Another veteran reflected his need to find positive meaning in the present, 'You forget the bad times, you don't dwell on the horror.' At the same time, this man had just discussed several bad experiences in a POW camp. So his meaning was related to the past, but defined in terms of where he was now. Others accepted the pain of the time without trying to cope, in the sense that they were not trying to remove the pain of the experience. Yet they were seeking some form of meaning. As one noted, 'You will never forget the look in a wounded man's eyes. You know, he's one of our team, they're hurting, you're hurting. That's why I said there's no humour in that moment.' Such statements were not made by everyone, which in part may reflect the incompleteness in this set of interview data, but it also reflects the nature of individual differences at any stage of life. Even in this small sample, not everyone felt the same way about their experiences.

Meaning can be defined in various ways. To Frankl, it involves a sense of purpose in the day-to-day activities of life, more so than seeking or finding any grand purpose (Frankl 1984). Peach (2003) uses a definition that sees spirituality as an experiential process that includes a quest for meaning and purpose, but he does not define meaning. Both meaning and spirituality are often regarded as part of the experience of being in the moment. Humour is also 'in the moment' and can be associated with the search for meaning, in that it highlights life's incongruities and absurdities. Yet humour (like spirituality) can help people transcend the moment. MacKinlay suggests that in later life, humour can be evidence of transcendence that arises in the process of life review, as well as a means to that transcendence (MacKinlay 2004).

For those who work in health and aged care, humour can be an end in itself, a pleasurable shared experience, and I accept we should not search for deep meaning in all humour. Sometimes something is just funny. However, I also propose that specific characteristics of humour can reveal a personal search for meaning and a sense of the spiritual dimension of life. This link is like a two-sided coin, which can be explained using the theories discussed previously in this chapter. For example, incongruity characteristic of humour can be linked to meaning at the level of the individual person; but it can also be linked to individual despair. Superiority aspects of humour can be linked to compassion, for example when we include ourselves in the joke; or to isolation, for example when we exclude ourselves or distance ourselves from others. Subversive humour can be associated with standing up for our values; but it can also be associated with despondency. The terms 'meaning', 'compassion', and 'values' are clearly part of most spiritual discussions, and when regarded in this light, humour can add to this spiritual dimension. But not all humour will do this. Much of the contemporary research work on humour and spirituality is still in its early stages, relying on surveys and very simple definitions of spirituality (if it is defined at all). It is obvious that people have long associated the two and will continue to do so, but more research, scholarship and informed speculation will help practitioners who wish to make concrete such a relationship and apply humour in their dealings with older clients.

Conclusion

This study provided an interesting window into veterans' views of humour in war. Today, that humour is of less concern to the veterans than reviewing stressful and demanding war experiences. The way the veterans focused on broad aspects of the past is characteristic of a later life search for meaning. It is possible (but not proven here) that the veterans were able to review their war experiences without traumatic symptoms because they had opened themselves to humour during war. Thus, short-term coping may, after all, have had some longer-term effect, even if just allowing the veterans to buy time and distance. Humour may have occasionally allowed them to access compassion, incongruity and interconnectedness in ways that were less painful than other direct ways. In this manner, humour may have helped them survive psychologically and spiritually to face their unpleasant experiences some decades later, with lesser threat to their well-being. For carers and health workers it may be useful to discuss this mixed role of humour with veterans.

The veterans chose not to highlight physical disabilities associated with ageing. Even though they did not use the term 'mental health', it seems they were more concerned to point out to us the previously unspoken challenges to mental health that were part of being a returned serviceman. Nevertheless, the findings here also have relevance to physical changes with ageing, as humour can enhance physical well-being to some degree (see Lefcourt 2001).

Similarly, humour can be used with those with deteriorating mental functioning. I was recently a participant at a laughter workshop in which most of the participants were older women from a dementia day care centre. It was a wonderful, funny and invigorating experience. At this stage, I wish to reiterate that sometimes humour can be of value just for its own sake. So regardless of whether this type of experience can be interpreted at a deeper level for meaning, or evaluated in a quantitative way, this type of humour-intervention was clearly of value in itself in terms of the obvious joy of all workshop participants. Joy may give meaning to life, as Frankl (1984) also observed.

MacKinlay (2004, p.44) has commented in her work on humour in later life: 'when I began my studies I did not seek to find instances of humour'. Yet she found humour in many of her participants' stories. As I have noted above, in this study we sought to find humour and found less than expected. Age does not make people identical, and people seek different approaches to their coping and resolution even when nominally in the same age group, such as later life. Humour may be one path to this resolution. Extreme experiences in early adulthood, such as war, contribute significantly to life review, and the search for resolution and meaning. The focus here was on veterans of the Second World War. Other cohorts of ageing veterans, for instance those of the Korean and Vietnam involvements, will have their own experiences which will add other dimensions to their stories. Letting people tell their versions, with informed assistance by health care workers, will allow us all to learn more about humour; finding meaning, and optimizing good mental health and well-being in later life.

Note

I wish to acknowledge the significant contribution of the late Margaret Massam.

CHAPTER 16

Pastoral Rituals, Ageing and New Paths into Meaning

Alan Niven

Three themes guide the content of this chapter for pastoral carers. The first is to observe and integrate the ritual patterns of your own life. The second is to develop an awareness of ritual processes. The third is to develop a facility with the practice of ritual.

Observing and integrating the ritual patterns of one's own life

> From beginning to end, the rituals of our lives shape each hour, each day, each year. Everyone leads a ritualized life: Rituals are repeated patterns of meaningful acts. If you are mindful of your actions, you will see the ritual patterns. If you see the patterns you may understand them. If you understand them, you may enrich them. In this way, the habits of a lifetime become sacred. Is this so? (Fulghum 1995, p.vi)

This chapter was developed from a 'hands-on' workshop with pastoral carers on the use of ritual in pastoral care. In order to catch the tone of the session, I will commence with a personal reflection on my pastoral formation within a Christian tradition, recognizing that there are similarities and differences to other faith traditions. I experience my mid-life journey of faith through the lens of Easter themes that prepare me for the next stage of the road. This lens has developed and guided my pastoral formation as I have responded to the reality of the practical signs and living symbols of death and resurrection that I experience in myself and others.

Nowadays it is difficult to define an actual age bracket and say 'that's mid-life' or 'that's where senior life begins', but there are some pivotal moments and inner-life activities that are common to this passage. I only have to consider the predictable and ordinary, celebratory or sad occasions that I and my circle of contemporaries have witnessed over the last decade: the silver wedding anniversaries of friends and the golden anniversaries of parents; the funerals of parents, favourite uncles, aunts, mentors and key figures from childhood and adolescence; the 21st parties of our children and their friends. The engagements of our children and their friends now remind us of our own distant celebrations; the act of helping married or partnered children move into new homes or watching the little arrivals tends to trigger strong memories; we ponder long and hard as our parents wave their final farewell to the family home; memorial or remembrance services bring many poignant reminders of mortality. This is life for me and the rest of the so-called sandwich generation. I am reminded that life consists of tiny points of connection that form stories that 'hold meaning only because of how someone hung them together... We do well to frame them – either literally, or by prayer, tears, stories, litanies of remembrance. Such mementoes matter a lot, especially when shared with loved ones' (Gibson and Gibson 1991, p.33).

Every celebration and ritual that I experience has a sketch of my dying to former patterns of living and a postcard from the future of my rising to new ways of being. The drive home or solitary moments in the garden the following day are often filled with seed-thoughts that are alternately sad and joyful, yet also convey the sense of a God who journeys with us. This represents for me an experience that is both strangely disturbing and comforting in its dual promise of struggle and hope.

An Easter-like theme emerges as I reflect upon my thoughts and feelings and I begin to connect with a truth or whisper of wisdom that has been a part of my spiritual journey: 'Very truly I tell you, unless a seed falls into the earth and dies, it remains just a single grain; but if it dies, it bears much fruit' (John 12:24 NRSV). Within my faith tradition this concept of relinquishing some aspect of my being provides one way of reframing loss, change and transition as a pathway to new and richer experiences.

When we pause to remember and pay attention to our own little deaths (or perhaps more literally those who have died), such moments may reveal great and small potholes of pain at our all-too-apparent frailties. We may also identify long-held regret over our mistakes and tugs of discomfort at our sins of omission. Even as this awareness trickles into our consciousness, one look in the mirror simultaneously reveals the brushstrokes of the years on our faces and again we confront our mortality. We may wish for one last conversation with those who have died or moved away. Perhaps we wish for a pen and a new page to write one more chapter with fewer mistakes. Questions begin to form. How will we live reflectively and engage new insights? How will we deal with the ripples from the past composed of the myriad triumphs and failures, neglected celebrations and accumulated grief from forgotten corners of our lives?

The predictable and continual appearance of these seed-moments offers fruitful times of reflection and self-awareness. One common factor becomes apparent. They are all usually accompanied by some form of ritual and in addition to 'the specific rituals of religious groups', it is important to affirm that 'rituals form an important aspect of life within any community' (MacKinlay 2006a, p.137). The diversity, richness and human dimension of ritual can serve to deepen our self-understanding and sensitivity to our own frameworks of faith and spiritual life. Such themes are shared with all humanity but for those of us who work in the caring professions, this reflection can also train us in the art of being open to ritual-making where the purpose of a ritual is to 'be cathartic, a way of releasing tension or pain…to invoke the presence of divinity or…to bridge the gulf between the human and physical world and the world of spirit and the unseen (Northcott 1993, p.191). As we observe our rituals and those of others in our family or community, we may well concur with psychiatrist and family researcher Jerry Lewis that if 'one wants to know what is central to a family's sense of its self, it may be best provided by a knowledge of the family rituals' (Lewis 1996, p.141). Lewis is simply affirming the insights of anthropology (Gennep 1909/1960; Turner 1969) that we will explore later in this chapter through the lens of pastoral theology.

The spiritual journey of mid-life, indeed the formation of pastoral carers, sometimes feels like the season of Easter with all its moments of preparation to accept the struggle, mercy and grace of God's own journey alongside our humanity. Whatever our faith perspective, this stage in the life-cycle prepares us for the tasks of later (perhaps sooner!) life where death and life confront us in even broader brushstrokes. Deeper growth in the light of these reflections may also continue to seep into our lives as we explore a mutuality in relationships where we can 'join [a] person in seeking revelation and believing that a way will open up that is not yet clearly seen' (Wicks and Rodgerson 1998, p.60). Our insights and discoveries are teased out in community, in conversation with peers and mentors or in robust exploration with supervisors and spiritual directors. Our experience of and reflection upon ritual is often the bridge to great self-discovery.

Evelyn and James Whitehead remind me that sadness, grief and ordinary (rather than clinical) depression can alert us that something has become intolerable. These passages of loss and seasons of regret 'invite us to re-examine our life; [their] misery motivates us to face a challenge or a loss we have been avoiding; it can ready us for mature grieving and change' (1995, p.7).

Mid-life and the later years prepare us for an appreciation of life and death in which the integration of losses and the celebration of new understanding emerge as a major theme. Loss, the journey through the life-cycle and the challenges of integrating our own experiences are very much a part of preparing to care for others. The daily round of life as a teacher in a context of pastoral formation, practical theology and theological field education leads me to observe in 20-, 30- and 40-year-olds similar patterns of growth and reflection to the ones that I experience in my 50s. I am very conscious of the relevance of McSherry's statement that spirituality 'is not a separate entity that can be turned on or off at the touch of a switch because it is continually present, whether we are conscious of this or not' (2006, p.89). McSherry argues that by 'fostering our own spiritual awareness we will be more focused and receptive to those who may have a spiritual concern' and hopefully, self-awareness generated through 'reflection, critical analysis and appraisal of oneself and experiences' can then add maturity and compassion to our service of others (p.164). I would add that the same is true of our ritual awareness. The challenge of integrating our own ritual experiences thus returns us to the wisdom of Fulghum. 'If you are mindful of your actions, you will see the ritual patterns. If you see the patterns you may understand them. If you understand them, you may enrich them' (1995, p.vi).

One of the goals of this chapter is to encourage carers to become more conscious of the role of ritual in their own lives if they wish to use or develop ritual as part of their pattern of care for others. Imber-Black and Roberts evaluate ritual from the perspective of the family therapist and raise a number of important questions (1992, pp.57–78). How will we identify where some crisis has interrupted sustaining rituals? How will we find the energy and courage to shift frozen rituals or challenge the obligatory rituals that oppress us and diminish our sense of self? What rituals have disappeared that we mourn or feel angry about? How do we critique the rigid rituals that rule our lives and which we no longer understand because their meaning has dissolved? I have become aware that if I can engage emotionally and cognitively in some sort of review of the rituals in my life (often with a supervisor or spiritual director) then my pastoral practice and sensitivity is enhanced accordingly. Imber-Black and Roberts suggest we start with ourselves:

> Whether the ritual style in your life now is minimized, interrupted, rigid, obligatory, imbalanced, or flexible, or some combination of these styles across various categories of rituals, you can examine your rituals and determine if they are meeting your relationship needs, or whether you want to try changing some of the patterns. (p.75)

This chapter argues that our facility with the use of ritual in a pastoral context, and our ability to explore the needs of others in a sensitive and creative way, is strongly linked to our own capacity for reflection. It matters little whether we simply use one Prayer Book and the same denominational resources all the time or create an eclectic pot-pourri from a variety of traditions or caring disciplines. However, it does matter what pastoral skills, professional safeguards and ritual theory we use to develop ritual responses to pastoral issues.

Developing an awareness of ritual processes

My early and ongoing formation in pastoral care owes much to writers who explored the theological and socio-political implications of ritual (Driver 1991; Moltmann 1977). While some writers engaged the pastoral application (Anderson and Foley 1998; Ramshaw 1987; Willimon 1979), others developed creative and inclusive rituals, prayers and responses (Abbott 2001; Goulart 2005; Ward and Wild 1995; Morley 1992). These writers and others have been my companions in pastoral conversation in response to the challenge of the suggestion that people

- are seeking to reinstate ritual as a source of spiritual identity, or collective action and belonging, and of personal and social transformation

- have taken up many of the functions and characteristics of ritual as it operated in primal, pre-modern cultures and re-engaged it with the quest for individual meaning and psychological well-being in the flux and melee of social and cultural life which represent the experience of modernity

- create rituals which reflect the smorgasbord character of the religious ideology and the symbol structure of the New Age, drawing upon many different spiritual paths and religious systems.

(Northcott 1993, pp.195–6)

It is now common for pastoral carers, myself included, to use careful listening skills and theological reflection in order to adjust the style, content, form and metaphors of any particular ritual to meet the needs, culture, context and wishes of the person or family. There has been for many years a greater willingness to move beyond the traditional, pre-constructed religious rituals while still valuing them as a core resource characterized by great beauty of form, theological insight and literary grace. Over twenty years ago, Ramshaw identified an important factor in the shifting nexus between formal communal ritual and an individualized pastoral creativity. The 'conflict many people see between ritual and an empathic response to individual needs has often been created by poor pastoral practice' (1987, p.55). One of the goals of pastoral formation has been to impart to students an understanding of good pastoral practice that 'involves both listening and praying, empathy and ritual' (p.56), and the false dichotomy between Ramshaw's 'ritualists' and 'counsellors' has thankfully dissolved. As a new pastor/counsellor in the late 1970s I appreciated William Willimon's (1979, p.17) cautionary reminder that C.S. Lewis said the charge was to 'feed my sheep' not 'run experiments on my rats'. With this warning in mind, a number of foundational factors have guided me over the years. They are common to any exploration of ritual theory but I owe my early integration of ritual within my pastoral practice to Moltmann's theology of hope in the context of ritual and worship (1977, pp.261–75).

Developing a facility with the practice of ritual

The discussion that follows seeks to develop a pastoral checklist that originates in a dialogue between theology and the social sciences that also incorporates the insights of pastoral theology and ritual theory.

Historical continuity (security)

Rituals serve as a buffer to the impact of the apparent speed and crisis of change and provide a sense of security when everything else seems to be disrupted or unstable. There is a predictable comfort in the regular visits of trusted persons, the reading of letters or a favourite book to a sight-impaired resident every Wednesday, and a quiet prayer or blessing offered at the end of a weekly service of worship. The observation of anniversaries, seasons, birthdays and times of remembrance help to regulate the rhythm of life and anticipate a future moment when the ritual will be enacted once more. As the past is engaged and brought into the present moment the participant in ritual often experiences a sense of ordering this future dimension, that in turn becomes what I would describe as a midwife to hope. Consider the words of Betty, frail and terminally ill, as she describes two rituals that sustain her – one obviously religious, the other a habit of a lifetime. 'My favourite magazine has arrived and Jean will be here soon to do the crossword with me. She writes the words in for me. I'm not enjoying the treatment at the moment but Jean and my crossword get me through.' MacKinlay highlights the value of ritual in an environment of aged care (2006a, p.137) and affirms Friedman's concept of 'orienting anchor' (2003, p.135). I have observed that people are desperately grateful for the 'anchor' effect of religious or long-term personal and social ritual as the emotional storms rage in a crisis, but it is also possible to become frozen or emotionally tied to one spot. The implication of 'orienting' suggests that effective or accurately-located ritual will enable a person to take a compass reading with a view to continuing their journey towards a yet-to-be-experienced horizon.

Betty went on to tell me about another important ritual. 'Our little worship service on a Friday is something I'd hate to miss. Even when I'm too sick to go I know they're praying for me. One day I won't be there at all, you know what I mean. That's ok. They'll still be there.' Betty has identified the two important rituals that sustain her in the present; one social, the other religious, but both deeply spiritual because they are linked to Betty's identity, sense of well-being and awareness of hope. She has also linked the traditions that have been a part of her life in the past (historical continuity) with her inner sense of peace about an unknown future. There is an element of personal commitment to the two rituals that have sustained her for many years. Her frailty has invited others in to share these special moments but the essence of personal hope continues to be expressed in each ritual. Betty's experience seems to indicate that a personal belief system and accompanying 'values and attitudes can bring hope in…the future or, from a religious perspective such as life everlasting, enabl[e] individuals to draw strength from their convictions and commitment' (McSherry 2006, p.56). Repetition is neither meaningless nor boring. Betty has made a choice, her present is linked to her past and her future is ordered – the rhythm of ritual has done its job. Effective carers will observe and take note.

Indicative character (meaning)

Ritual therefore 'invites us to remembrance, to hope, or to a new page in life' that may even be prompted by our anticipated death (Moltmann 1977, p.263), and through this process, continually serves to affirm and reaffirm meaning (Friedman 2003, p.135). Relevance in the present emerges because the ritual becomes the symbol that points beyond itself. However, the ritual must be interpreted within the culture and family system to which it belongs or from which it develops. 'What we have grown up with is both familiar and will be the vehicle of meaning for us. To be deprived of this may be particularly distressing' (MacKinlay 2006a, p.136). My partner-discipline of family therapy has reinforced for me the need to engage people in pastoral conversation on this topic as I seek to offer care prior to exploration of the use of ritual, whether pre-constructed or yet to be created. 'Taking some time to tell stories about previous rituals is another way to draw people into the process of ritual reflection, and ultimately broader participation' (Imber-Black and Roberts 1992, p.294). It is neither appropriate nor advisable to use this approach with all people but I need to be informed and guided by people's stories and open to all possibilities, or the end result may be more about *my* meaning rather than the resident's or parishioner's meaning. Consider the ritual of prayer. Ramshaw's description of the tension that existed, and still exists, for the carer is helpful:

> The split between 'ritualists' and 'counsellors' has gone so deep that, at the other extreme from the unempathic ritualist, one finds the [carer] who listens and listens and never prays. This may be appropriate in some situations…but as a constant strategy it can be just as much a means of avoidance as unasked-for ritualising. (1987, p.56)

I suspect that clergy or chaplains in the past may have felt that the task of ritual-making belonged exclusively to them and perhaps they even believed that discussion on the topic might be too much for the resident or parishioner. This is why I was talking to Betty in the first place. She became my instructor in her world of meaning, symbol and ritual as together we prepared a small service in which she would hand over her rings (wedding and engagement) to her two daughters. I outline the case study below.

A case study – the two rings

Betty is 89 and a widow. Her husband died many years ago and until her fall she lived independently. She has two daughters who live nearby and one son interstate. The daughters provide excellent care through visiting and companionship – the three of them are, in effect, very good friends. Betty wants to sell her house and find a permanent home that suits her level of health. In the last three months other complicating illnesses have developed and Betty's doctor has indicated that Betty may not 'get through'. One daughter is very realistic and asks for information but the other does not really want to face the facts and keeps insisting that mum will one day go home. For Betty, each day becomes a difficult journey of adjusting to the two perspectives of her daughters. Her honest talks with her doctor have revealed to her what she suspected. She is failing rapidly and her doctor is talking in terms of months. One daughter refuses to acknowledge this and the other, who accepts the situation and talks to her mother about it, is becoming more frustrated as the days go by.

> Betty talks to you as her pastoral carer. She wants to pass her rings on to her daughters, hoping that the meaning will be apparent for the one who is struggling. She asks you to pray as she does this. You have taken this conversation on to the point where she sees the value of a small service/ritual. Betty has a realistic, practical and firm faith. She attends the Chapel service when she can and she misses her local church. The daughters do not express their faith overtly or attend church but they respect, value and support their mother's faith. Betty wants you to 'run' the service and says 'You'll know what to do. I've thought about it a lot since we talked and I'm so worried about my daughter. I think it will help her. You know I'll be saying goodbye, don't you, and this is the only way I can?'

The inherent questions raised by this case study revolve around some of the issues noted below:

- How do I negotiate the power I have been given? How do I best use Betty's trust?

- To what extent do I seek to involve the daughters as we work on the service? If the 'planning time that precedes a ritual can be as important as the ritual itself' (Imber-Black and Roberts 1992, p.83), how do I work with the obvious love and intimacy that already exists between these three women?

- No matter how much trust I have been given, how much is the carer or pastor always a *welcome stranger* who walks on holy ground?

- Should I seek to confront the issues directly or will we run with the mother's less confrontational approach, let the ritual do its work and then see what develops?

- All rituals need some sort of statement of purpose. What is the purpose of this ritual and who will articulate this? If ritual is the symbol that points beyond itself, what is the meaning that 'becomes present in an accentuated way'? (Moltmann 1977, p.264)

A ritual framework incorporates social significance

Friedman's 'orienting anchor' also owes much to a sense of participation that is enhanced by the reduction of isolation and the building of community. Moltmann affirms that every ritual 'stands in a framework of social coherences and also establishes social coherences' (1977, p.264) in such a way that changes in our role and identity can be marked. In other words, as people observe our rituals they see who we are or are becoming, our character is expressed and our belief systems portrayed. In ritual

> all take their parts in a collective dance or drama – it involves an inner consent and an outer submission to the forms and rhythms of the rite... Ritual also involves the breaking of the usual boundaries and hierarchies of social life – what Victor Turner calls the liminal moment where identities are fused and social status is temporarily abrogated. (Northcott 1993, p.191)

There are three phases to this process: separation, liminality, reincorporation (Gennep 1909/1960; Turner 1969; Driver 1991, pp.157–65).

Separation

In this phase, symbolic behaviour signifies the detachment of the individual or group. In a marriage ceremony a couple about to be married will move away from their family of origin and their parents in particular, often with some gesture of recognition that the moment is symbolic of *leaving and cleaving*. The young scout, prior to his investiture with badges of graduation, will cross a symbolic river to stand apart from the pack. Similarly, the worker recently made redundant is invited to come forward in the lunchroom and receive a gift from his peers after clearing his tools from the workshop and washing up. Betty comes out from the daily life of her aged care community to join a small group of fellow worshippers.

Liminality

During this phase, the characteristics of the subject are ambiguous because they are in a process of change or transition. They are neither one thing nor the other. People stand on the threshhold (Latin *limen*) of a new role, identity or, in Betty's daughter's case, a new understanding of her relationship with her mother. During the ritual we have left the past and we do not yet have the attributes, insights or awareness of our future state. The bride and groom in a wedding service pause in that pre-celebratory space before they are announced to be husband and wife. The scout stands with his badges but has not yet stepped back to rejoin his awaiting peers and enact among them his new privileges. The worker stands before his peers as he prepares to leave his workplace, acknowledges the gift as a parting symbol of what they have shared together and speaks a few words about what he may see as the future.

In fact it was at the pivotal point in our ritual of the two rings (as they were taken off and handed over) that Betty's daughter began to cry. The whole experience in her mother's hospital room had seemed what she described as 'surreal' until that moment when the meaning dawned. Of course the insights had been kept locked down by denial and conspired with the movements of the ritual to create an atmosphere where she felt 'something was about to happen'. The 'something' was the arrival of a truth where her tears of present and anticipatory grief were met by the embrace of her mother and sister as they comforted her. The daughter still has to move on from this liminal point and live in her new state of being.

Reincorporation

The rite of passage or ritual is consummated, the subject is now redefined in a new state with fresh rights and obligations. Identified and introduced as husband and wife the couple walk forward to be greeted, welcomed and accepted into their community in a new role. The scout rejoins his peers and exercises his new status. The newly retired worker moves out of the workplace, conscious that he no longer belongs to the group and leaves as a member of society with a different role. Betty's daughter begins to live in a world where she is confronted with the reality that her mother will not be with her in the same ways she has known.

What is the significance of our own story for our reflective practice? I wonder, if as we stand at the liminal, transitional, feeling-filled and intense moment between separation and reincorporation at many points in our lives (often crisis points and rites of passage), we are at our most individuated because we do not know to whom we belong, who we are or how we will cope. Hopefully our reflection will lead us to deal more wisely and sensitively with those in our care as we remember in glimpses of mutuality the vulnerability, fragility and paradox of those moments.

The 'human' purposes of ritual

One of the reflective questions I often use in supervision sessions is specifically related to lifelong experience of ritual: 'How do the rituals in your life work for you?' The discussion will then be based on a number of differentiating themes as we focus on rituals that address *relating, changing, healing, believing* and *celebrating* (Imber-Black and Roberts 1992, pp. 26–56). I then invite the student to identify and critique key issues where their own experience can inform and critique their own practice.

Relating

Rituals can give us the opportunity to shape, express and maintain relationships. We then discuss the major life-cycle shifts and identify what rituals worked or didn't work.

Changing

As we go through transitions we use rituals to create and indicate for ourselves and others the changes we are accepting or grappling with. I invite the student to identify the emotional, spiritual and practical support they received and ask them to apply the insights to a case study from their own practice.

Healing

Rituals can facilitate the recovery process after loss, times of trauma or relationship breakdown. I invite the student to write up a story of some form of healing they have experienced. We work together to identify the people, places, times and seasons, and then identify any ritual or liturgical aspects. In the case of chaplains or pastoral carers, theological reflection will lead us to consider biblical and theological insights and resources.

Believing

Rituals are ways of expressing and giving voice to life beliefs even as we explore the meaning of that belief. 'One of the functions of ritual is to mark the pathways for morality to follow' (Driver 1991, p.33). I invite the student to reflect on the meaning for them of aspects of ritual such as prayer, blessings, anointing, listening as faithful companioning, presence, silence, touch, the sacred, or communion. Once again I am grateful to the wisdom of Fulghum: 'If you are mindful of your actions, you will see the ritual patterns... In this way, the habits of a lifetime become sacred' (1995, p.vi). I then ask the student to write up a ritual they have used and identify the contours and shapes of belief even as they consider the value of being alert to their ritual selves.

Celebrating

Rituals provide us with the opportunity to affirm and recognize with joy and thanksgiving all aspects of our lives. Strangely this is a theme that many students find difficult. It is satisfying when they begin to apprehend dimensions of thanksgiving in the simple rituals of sleep, restored health, a walk with the dog, a meal on the table, employment or even a completed assignment! Shopping, mowing the lawn, hospital visiting, reading or writing *become* the stuff of ritual that enables us to celebrate who we are. I have observed that exploration of this theme enables carers to develop rituals that flow naturally and unselfconsciously out of the ordinary. Whether the pastoral carer uses a prayer book or a poetry book, a pre-constructed ritual or a collaborative gem, the people they care for seem to dwell comfortably in the meaning and flow of the ritual.

The reality of pastoral power

How do we communicate with each other in ritual-making? There is often a power crisis as we develop skills in this area. Many years ago I enjoyed applying Habermas' concepts of communicative competence (1981, pp.325–9) to my church roles and wider community pastoral roles. Effective ritual-makers will engage and embody the following four characteristics:

1. Each person has a roughly equal opportunity to speak and contribute from their particular perspective. How often does this happen when someone approaches a minister or a priest, a pastoral carer or a celebrant?

2. There is a balanced subject or object role during the dynamics of interaction. This is seen in the ability to influence events such as choice of ritual, decisions on time and place and as to whether or not the various parties are free to participate. Is it truly a collaborative exercise?

3. A symmetry of complementary modes is demonstrated e.g. speaking and listening, questioning and answering, concealing and revealing. This will indicate whether or not they even connect with us as human beings. How mutual is the encounter and who has control?

4. The same rules and norms apply to all participants and no participant has any privileged position. We can only speak of each person being valued for their unique contribution to the process. There is nothing wrong with one person having more experience, education or expertise but are the dynamics expressive of values we cherish such as equality, shalom, freedom of expression or justice-making?

Let me tell you what happened with Betty's ritual. She had begun by saying 'you'll know what to do'. The process concluded with Betty choosing the readings and prayers from selections I brought, organizing a private space with the nurse, ordering afternoon tea for us all and deciding exactly how she would hand over the rings and what she would say. She asked my advice on some aspects of grief and asked me to open the time with a statement of purpose that we drew up together. I also closed with a prayer and a blessing as mother and daughters held hands with each other. I was very conscious of being a privileged guest. Consider also the dynamics of the following case study where another face of power becomes apparent – the hierarchy of caregivers that sometimes inhibits the community of caregivers.

A case study in sharing power

I received a phone call one Saturday morning from a nurse (Paul) in an aged care facility close to the college where I teach. He explained that James was dying and asked me to come and pray. He explained that he had known James a number of years and James had asked him to ensure that prayers would be offered at the end of his life. However no minister was available and his remaining family lived interstate. I told Paul I would come. When I arrived I saw that he had placed a screen around the bed, and a table was laid with a white cloth and an open Bible. Flowers had been set up, a cassette recorder was playing sacred music and a candle had been lit. James had obviously just had his hair combed, his breathing was erratic and the doctor had just left. Paul was obviously fond of his elderly patient but when I arrived he explained the context again and quietly prepared to withdraw. I asked if he would like to stay. He nodded, drew the curtains and waited. I began to open the books I had brought and asked if he would like to read one of the passages of Scripture. He paused and then nodded so I also indicated one of the prayers that focused on God's continuing care for James. 'Is that ok?' he asked. 'If you would like to' I replied. In the end we shared the ritual. Paul read Scripture, prayed and assisted me in a simple service, as James quietly took his final breaths.

I felt that our companionship created a sense of community that embraced James. I wondered about other occasions when through busyness, insecurity, insensitivity or tiredness I may have lost the opportunity for what Turner (1969) described as the twin concepts of *liminality* and *communitas*. These concepts denote moments when ritual serves to diffuse hierarchy, equalize power, bring unity and level social structure. A number of questions emerged from this incident. How would I describe my role? Who should be the facilitator of the ritual? How often do those with pastoral power assume the compliance of others without really thinking? How does the role of the 'expert' diminish the level of care that we offer? What are the systemic and cultural issues that collude with the way we use power? I could ask many more questions but Driver sums up my thoughts. 'Ritual is the license we give one another and our spirituality to don bright colours and move in circles and claim this moment as kairos. Only where there is death does ritual cease. Without it we literally die' (1991, p.9).

Practical guidelines

I have found the insights of other carers invaluable. Early writers on ritual and pastoral care (Renner 1979; Willimon 1979) enabled me to develop an inner checklist as I explored pastoral issues with parishioners and residents. I discovered similar themes in Mitchell (1989) and the following themes incorporate some of his pastoral insights.

1. Discuss the issue with all parties and perhaps just 'imagine' for a while.

2. Think of others who could perform or participate in the ritual. While respecting the role of appropriate 'experts' remember that life experiences or special relationships may be qualifications that we sometimes neglect.

3. Allow the stories and metaphors of each person to be offered and valued. Within this context enable those involved to work collaboratively with you in the design of the ritual.

4. You may give guidance on the form but it is good to enable others to develop, draft and design the content.

5. Remember that any ritual may have many different and significant meanings for each person involved. A similar issue may occur for other parties but meaning is not necessarily transferable.

6. For those whose practice on a one-on-one basis prompts the use of ritual, it is important to be cautious. Community rituals or those involving a number of people have fewer inherent risks and more checks and balances.

7. The reality of pastoral boundaries and incidents of abuse have challenged the ministry of touch but careful practice and rituals such as anointing or blessing are valuable resources.

8. As I have already noted there has been for many years a greater willingness to move beyond traditional, pre-constructed religious rituals. We must still value them as a core resource characterized by great beauty of form, theological insight and literary grace.

Conclusion

I leave the final words to Robert Fulghum's Propositions on Ritual.

- To be human is to be religious
- To be religious is to be mindful
- To be mindful is to pay attention
- To pay attention is to sanctify existence
- Rituals are one way in which attention is paid
- Rituals arise from the ages and stages of life
- Rituals transform the ordinary into the holy
- Rituals may be public, private or secret
- Rituals may be spontaneous or arranged
- Rituals are constantly evolving and reforming
- Rituals create sacred time
- Sacred time is the dwelling place of the eternal
- Haste and ambition are the adversaries of sacred time. Is this so?

(1995, p.20)

CHAPTER 17

Ageing, Disability and Spirituality: The Possibilities for Well-being and Care

Elizabeth MacKinlay

In this final chapter I will reflect on some of the questions raised by the audience for the panel at the conclusion of the conference. Further, I will address directions for future practice and research in the fields of ageing, disability and spirituality. This book has provided a number of perspectives on ageing, disability and spirituality. It is our hope that readers who engage with the material presented in these chapters may be challenged to radical new ways of being, in relationships, care and advocacy for older people with disabilities. Not all of the material presented is new, but taken together, it challenges the ethos of policy-makers and organizations, including the church, that provide services and care for disabled and older people.

At the end of the conference there was a call from the conference participants for substantial changes to be made to the structure and presentation of services and care for older people with disabilities. It was affirmed during the conference that for too long, pastoral care has been an optional component of care; the time has now come to bring pastoral and spiritual care into the body of knowledge and practice of care providers. A media release from the conference called for the establishment of a taskforce to examine the role of pastoral and spiritual care within aged care and to set standards for care and education for pastoral care. There are already structures in place through the standards set by the Aged Care Standards and Accreditation Agency for Australia. However, the guidelines do not in any clear way set out what constitutes spiritual care in ageing. The extent to which it is set out in the guidelines is to note that spiritual and cultural needs should be met. The Aged Care Standards (3.8) require attention to culture and spirituality, but how do we do it? Other standards perhaps implicitly relate to spirituality: Standard 1 is needed to provide the basis on which to give appropriate care. Standard 2 is also important, and 2.8, pain management as well as 2.9, palliative care, are especially relevant to spiritual needs, but these standards are often interpreted to include care other than spiritual. There is a real need to provide guidelines that can inform practice.

Although 'spirituality' has become a buzz word in the wider community, and more is being written about spirituality, much of this writing has little of value to guide practice. Some schools of medicine and nursing are teaching spiritual care; the content is often very ad hoc. In numbers of academic and practice settings, there is still confusion over the differences between religion and spirituality. There are few courses in pastoral care and ageing in Australia, apart from the courses offered through the Centre for Ageing and Pastoral Studies. As yet, there has been little attempt to structure pastoral and spiritual care, or to incorporate spiritual care into aged care generally.

At the same time there is a growing literature on spirituality in health care, from medicine (Koenig 1998), nursing (Swinton 2001; McSherry 2006; MacKinlay 2006b) and social work (Moody 2005). Some of this is related to spirituality in ageing, yet the research is still in its infancy in providing a firm basis for practice. Further research is needed to examine how spiritual care sits within the practice of existing health professions.

In aged care, in particular, it seems reasonable to consider spiritual care as being part of diversional therapy, and it may be easier to incorporate spiritual care into this new and developing professional discipline than into established professions. Nursing and medicine, I suggest, need to reflect much more deeply on what form spiritual care should take in these professions, as their practice areas and boundaries are more firmly set. I note that spiritual care does not adjust easily to prescribing treatments. It is more likely to become incorporated into psychological care, as there are already paradigms for psychological strategies and care. Much of the research so far, particularly from the USA, has been conducted by researchers from within this discipline. I see a tendency to simply add spirituality to the existing psychological care and a failure to recognize that spiritual care, although closely associated with psychological care, has quite distinct areas of concern. Therefore further research into spirituality and spiritual care must be undertaken, not as an adjunct to existing scientific paradigms, but as an entity in its own right. Should this not be undertaken, it will be to the detriment of the needs for spiritual care. The work of Swinton and Mowat (2006) is an important way forward into appropriate ways of researching spirituality and chaplaincy. They make the strong link between practical theology and qualitative research and it is only as we more deeply examine the phenomena of spirituality that we will find the ways forward.

Some of the research reported on in this book has used such qualitative methods of inquiry (Ceramidas, MacKinlay, Robertson-Gillam). At this stage of development of our knowledge of spirituality, we need to keep asking the people whose lives are central to our work and study: What does this mean for you? How is spirituality important in your life? How can we assist you? Even when we may think that the person does not have a voice, as too frequently happens for people with dementia and other mental disabilities, we should never make that assumption. For example, we found that people with significant dementia could still contribute in valuable ways to assisting us build up our knowledge of their spiritual needs (MacKinlay, Trevitt and Coady 2002–2005).

Dementias

How do we move into the future in caring more effectively for people with dementia? Apart from the magic cure that seems to continue to recede into the future, there needs to be hope for people with dementia now. Chapters in this book have dealt with a number of important issues relating to dementia care, from Swinton's emphasis on personhood and theology to McNamara's ethical perspective on disability. Goldsmith's chapter considers suffering and dementia; Bryden wrote as she struggled with progressing fronto-temporal dementia, while Robertson-Gillam's work uses choir with people who have depression and some with dementia, where an intervention within aged care facilities has opened up new ways of finding meaning for these people. We continue to advocate for the well-being of people with dementia. We continue to research, not just for the magic cure, but for ways of improving the quality of life for people with dementia. Hughes, Louw and Sabat see the importance of language and sharing in speech in the public space.

> It is when the public space breaks down in dementia because of the loss of the 'shared life-world', that meaning-making becomes difficult. The reaction, however, should not be to abandon the enterprise of trying to communicate, but to look for new interpretations (in line with hermeneutics) in order to re-create the shared public space insofar as this is possible; but it should not be assumed that this will be impossible, only that it might require effort. (2006, p.23)

Hope for the future is to be found in statements such as these; this is as Kitwood (1997) has said in the past – the onus is on the person without dementia to reach out in communication to the person with dementia. This is echoed in the words of Hughes *et al.* (2006, p.26):

> It follows that not only does the person with dementia retain aspects of their personhood in and through those around, but also that those caring for the person retain their humanity in remaining engaged with and exercising respect for the person who relies upon them for their care.

This is a message that must be spread widely, through the community and among aged care workers, churches and policy-makers. A change of heart and attitudes is needed, to realize that not only do those with dementia need those who do not have dementia, but also, and just as importantly, those of us who do not have dementia need those who have it.

Woods (2005) notes that as we look to the future and the expected increases in the prevalence of dementia in the community, greater understanding is needed as to why some people can continue to function well despite the presence of brain pathology (p.258). He asks what factors may be modifiable. He also notes the real difficulty in maintaining people with dementia at home in the long term, even with packages of community care. These are certainly areas to be examined from the viewpoint of pastoral community care.

Engaging in the ministry of being with and caring for older people

Responses from the panel to this question of 'how do we do it?' acknowledged that this ministry is broader than the residential aged care community. The community extends out into the wider community, and especially the community of faith from which the person came. Rosalie Hudson told a story that clearly illustrates the lack of seeing beyond the walls of institutions in some cases.

She told of an elderly woman who was moving to residential care. This woman was farewelled and a presentation given to her in recognition of her gifts and service in the congregation by her community of faith before she moved. The irony was that she was moving to a hostel just around the corner from her church. Yet, there was a clear and definite separation between the two communities. There are numbers of communities where real linkages exist between residential aged care and the communities outside of the institution; more are needed. While aged care ministry requires special skills and education in an ageing society, greater awareness of the needs of older people is needed by the wider community as well. There are ways of promoting the connections between community and the aged care facility. In some cases, teams of pastoral carers maintain links with the aged care facilities in their areas, providing regular visiting and services that support the work of the chaplains.

Too often there are shortages of chaplains who have completed study in ageing and pastoral care, leaving those in need of care with less than adequate care to support their pastoral and spiritual needs.

What is a healthy church?

This question came to the panel from conference participants, and it related to some comments critical of attitudes towards older people, and especially those with disabilities, for instance, the comment of Newell:

> All around the world church leaders talk piously of the importance of healthy churches and the easy solutions to life provided you follow their ten-point plan. I can but suggest that life is sacred not despite disability, but also through the woundedness we all share as persons.

The panel response that really answered this question came from Eileen Glass as she affirmed that the healthy church is an inclusive church. She went on to describe the healthy church as being a place where every member had a place, illustrated by St Paul, writing of the parts of the body (1 Corinthians 12:14–26); each needing the other. She said:

> For me, one of the most profound things that he says in that text about the eye, is that the eye is not the ear and the hand is not the foot, and so on. He says it is precisely those parts of the body which seem the weakest that are the indispensable ones. And until we know how to have a conversation about indispensable weakness and indispensable vulnerability, that is, the reality of limitation as part of who we are, I don't think we will be building a healthy church.

There is a tendency in some churches to have different services that attract different groups of people, for instance, more traditional services are held and more often older people will attend, while more informal types of worship services seem to appeal to younger people. While this may nicely meet the needs of the different age groups, it leads to a separation of people from each other. It is therefore important to intentionally encourage linkages between the age groups within communities of faith. Both the young and the old of the community need each other and have much to both give and receive from each other. Disabilities, of course, go right across the lifespan; we have simply targeted older people who have disabilities in this selection of essays. It is also important that all people, disabled and non-disabled, are enabled to become authentic parts of the community of faith. We all, collectively, comprise the Body of Christ.

How can care practices be changed?

Care practices will not be changed unless we can demonstrate a firm base of knowledge and models for care in the fields of pastoral and spiritual care. Why do I use both these terms? I see pastoral care in the same terms as nursing care: it is about a specific type of care. Pastoral care has a long tradition as a modality of care. At one level, it means journeying with a person, on a one-to-one relationship. It assumes at least a basic level of training in human relationships, a basic theological background, and a sound understanding of oneself as the provider of care. Spiritual care is the type of care of the spirit that may be provided by different health care providers, through, for example, medicine, nursing or social care. Spiritual care is then one part of the practice of these health care providers.

Care practices will change when the benefits of providing spiritual and pastoral care can be demonstrated, with observed outcomes of care. For changes to policy and structures of care to occur, these demonstrated outcomes will need to be related to cost-effectiveness. Currently, it is easier to demonstrate outcomes through quantative research. Spirituality does not fit neatly into boxes, and is more difficult to measure objectively. However, the increasing rigour of qualitative research methods will make it easier to show changes.

We are back to research again. It is almost a chicken and egg situation. We cannot make substantial changes in spiritual care unless we can show evidence of improved outcomes of care. We don't know if our spiritual care makes a difference, so we turn to research. We cannot get the types of answers we need through quantative research. Qualitative research methods do allow us to ask the right questions, and further, allow the participants of research to name their questions, so that this research is more likely to be participant-driven, rather than driven by the agendas of the researchers. However, the findings of qualitative research are not well accepted by the scientific community. Therefore it is difficult to change practice. In the meantime, there are many places where dedicated carers do provide effective pastoral and spiritual care, with little support. Often it is 'going the extra mile' rather than being a part of one's role. Or, pastoral care may be done by volunteers, valuable volunteers; but nevertheless, the work of these people has not been valued enough to warrant paying them.

Conclusion: future directions in pastoral and spiritual care

The body of knowledge and understanding of the discipline of pastoral care, and the growing inclusion of spiritual care into allied health-care-provider education and practice, justifies establishment of suitable preparation in these fields.

Research is proliferating in nursing, medicine and social work, as well as in other health-related fields, and more of it is using qualitative methods. Diversional therapists also claim some role in spiritual care. The time is ripe for considering roles of the respective health care providers, in relation to their existing roles. The chaplaincy role in ageing, religion and spirituality is a specialty role. And yet, this role too is changing within the context of changing societies, and the need to address issues of increasingly multicultural and multifaith communities.

In this book, we have raised important issues related to the themes of ageing, disability and spirituality. We have called for serious attention to the ways of caring for and affirming older and disabled people, as equally valuable people in our communities. We have challenged the dominant values of individualism and autonomy and called for recognition of our needs for interdependency, both of disabled people with others and for non-disabled people with those who are disabled. As we continue on the journey, there is much that disabled and non-disabled people can learn from each other.

References

Abbott, M. (2001) *Sparks of the Cosmos: Rituals for Seasonal Use.* Adelaide: MediaCom.

Achenbaum, W.A. and Modell, S.M. (1999) 'Joan and Erik Erikson and Sarah and Abraham: Parallel Awakenings in the Long Shadow of Wisdom and Faith.' In L.E. Thomas and S.A. Eisenhandler (eds) *Religion, Belief, and Spirituality in Late Life.* New York, NY: Springer.

Alexopolous, G.S., Abrams, R.C., Young, R.C. and Shamoian, C.A. (1988) 'Cornell scale for depression in dementia.' *Biological Psychiatry 23,* 3, 271–84.

Alzheimer's Australia (2003) *The Dementia Epidemic: Economic Impact and Positive Solutions for Australia.* Canberra: Access Economics Pty Ltd.

Alzheimer's Australia (2004) *Dementia Terminology Framework: Position Paper 4.* Canberra: Alzheimer's Australia.

Alzheimer's Disease International (2006) '100 years of Alzheimer's Disease: No Time to Lose!' *Global Perspective 16,* 1, 1.

American Psychiatric Association (1994) *Diagnostic and Statistical Manual of Mental Disorders: DSM-IV.* Washington, DC: APA.

Anderson, A. (2002) 'Treatment of Depression in Older Adults.' *International Journal of Psychosocial Rehabilitation 6,* 69–78.

Anderson, H. and Foley, E. (1998) *Mighty Stories, Dangerous Ritual.* San Francisco, CA: Jossey-Bass.

Anderson, N.T. (1990) *Victory over the Darkness: Realizing the Power of Your Identity in Christ.* Ventura, CA: Regal Books.

Anderson, N.T. (1993) *The Bondage Breaker.* Eugene, OR: Harvest House.

Atkinson, D.V. and Field, D.H. (eds) (1995) *New Dictionary of Christian Ethic and Pastoral Theology.* Leicester: Inter-Varsity Press.

Austin, D. (2001) 'In Search of the Self: The Use of Vocal Holding Techniques with Adults Traumatized as Children.' *Music Therapy Perspectives 19,* 22–30.

Australian Bureau of Statistics (1998) *Mental Health and Wellbeing: Profile of Adults, Australia, 1997.* Canberra: ABS.

Australian Bureau of Statistics (2004a) *Australian Social Trends, 2004.* Canberra: ABS.

Australian Bureau of Statistics (2004b) *Population by Age and Sex, Australia.* Canberra: ABS.

Australian Bureau of Statistics (2004c) *Disability, Ageing and Carers, Australia: Summary of Findings (2003).* Accessed on 15 March 2007 at: www.abs.gov.au/AUSSTATS/abs@.nsf/mf/4430.0?OpenDocument

Australian Institute of Health and Welfare (1997) *The Definition of Disability in Australia: Moving towards National Consistency.* Accessed on 15 March 2007 at: www.aihw.gov.au/publications/index.cfm/title/95

Australian Institute of Health and Welfare (2000a) *Disability and Ageing: Australian Population Patterns and Implications.* Canberra: AIHW.

Australian Institute of Health and Welfare (2000b) *Residential Aged Care Facilities in Australia 1998–99: A Statistical Overview.* Accessed on 15 March 2007 at: www.aihw.gov.au/publications/welfare/racfa98-9/index.html

Baroody, K. (2006) Circular Letter.

Barrett, J. (1995) *We Were There.* St Leonards, NSW: Allen and Unwin (Penguin Edition).

Beck, A.T. (1967) *Depression.* New York, NY: Hoeber.

Becker, A.H. (1986) *Ministry with Older Persons: A Guide for Clergy and Congregations.* Minneapolis, MN: Ausburg Publishing House.

Bianchi, E.C. (1992) *Aging as a Spiritual Journey.* New York, NY: Crossroad.

Bigby, C. (2004) *Ageing with a Lifelong Disability: A Guide to Practice, Program, and Policy Issues for Human Services Professionals.* London: Jessica Kingsley Publishers.

Bird, M. and Luszcz, M. (1993) 'Enhancing Memory Performance in Alzheimer's Disease: Acquisition Assistance and Cue Effectiveness.' *Journal of Clinical and Experimental Neuropsychology 15*, 6, 921–32.

Blazer, D.G., Sachs-Ericsson, N. and Hybels, C.F. (2005) 'Perception of Unmet Basic Needs as a Predictor of Mortality among Community-Dwelling Older Adults.' *American Journal of Public Health 95*, 2, 299–304.

Blazer, H., Hughes, D. and George, L. (1987) 'The Epidemiology of Depression in an Elderly Community Population.' *The Gerontologist 27*, 281–87.

Boden, C. (1998) *Who Will I Be When I Die?* Pymble: Harper Collins Religious.

Bonhoeffer, D. (1978 [1966]) *Christ the Center,* trans. J. Bowden from the German *Christologie* (in *Gesammelte Schriften III*, 166–242). New York, NY: Harper & Row.

Bonhoeffer, D. (1998) *Sanctorum Communio: A Theological Study of the Sociology of the Church,* trans. R. Krauss and N. Lukens; ed. C. Green. Minneapolis, MN: Fortress.

Book of Common Prayer (1662) *The Order of the Administration of the Lord's Supper.* Fourth collect to be said after the offertory when there is no communion.

Bowker, J. (1997) *The Oxford Dictionary of World Religions.* New York, NY: Oxford University Press.

Boyd, J.W. (1986) 'Suffering in Theravada Buddhism.' In K.N. Tiwari (ed.) *Suffering: Indian Perspectives.* New Delhi: Motilal Banarsidass, 145–62.

Brodie, T. (2001) *Genesis as Dialogue: A Literary, Historical, and Theological Commentary.* Oxford: Oxford University Press.

Brueggemann, W. (1999) *The Covenanted Self: Explorations in Law and Covenant.* Minneapolis, MN: Fortress.

Brussat, F. and Brussat, M.A. (1996) *Spiritual Literacy: Reading the Sacred in Everyday Life.* New York, NY: Touchstone.

Bryden, C. (2005) *Dancing with Dementia: My Story of Living Positively with Dementia.* London: Jessica Kingsley Publishers.

Burnside, I. (1995) 'Themes and Props: Adjuncts for Reminiscence Therapy Groups.' In B.K. Haight and J.D. Webster (eds) *The Art and Science of Reminiscing: Theory, Research, Methods, and Applications.* Washington, DC: Taylor and Francis.

Butler, R., Lewis, M. and Sunderland, T. (1991) *Aging and Mental Health: Positive Psychological and Biomedical Approaches.* Columbus, OH: Charles Merrill.

Charmaz, K. (2003) 'Qualitative Interviewing and Grounded Theory Analysis.' In J.A. Holstein and J.F. Gubrium (eds) *Inside Interviewing: New Lenses, New Concerns.* Thousand Oaks, CA: Sage.

Clair, A. (2000) 'The Importance of Singing with Elderly Patients.' In D. Aldridge (ed.) *Music Therapy in Dementia Care.* London: Jessica Kingsley Publishers, 81–101.

Clarke, D. (2003) 'Faith and Hope.' *Australasian Psychiatry 11,* 2, 164–8.

Clements, W.M. (ed.) (1981) *Ministry with the Aging: Designs, Challenges, Foundations.* Cambridge: Harper and Row.

Clendinnen, I. (2001) *Tiger's Eye: A Memoir.* London: Jonathan Cape.

Close, R.E. (2000) 'Logotherapy and Adult Major Depression: Psychotheological Dimensions in Diagnosing the Disorder.' In M.A. Kimble (ed.) *Viktor Frankl's Contribution to Spirituality and Aging.* New York, NY: Haworth Press.

Coleman, P.G. (1999) 'Creating a Life Story: The Task of Reconciliation.' *The Gerontologist 39,* 2, 133–9.

Coleman, P.G., McKiernan, F., Mills, M. and Speck, P. (2002) 'Spiritual Belief and Quality of Life: The Experience of Older Bereaved Spouses.' *Quality in Ageing – Policy, Practice and Research 3,* 1, 20–26.

Commonwealth of Australia (1992) *Disability Discrimination Act 1992.*

Commonwealth of Australia (2002) *Intergenerational Report 2002–03,* Budget Paper No. 5. Canberra: CoA.

Commonwealth of Australia (2006) *Guidelines for a Palliative Approach in Residential Aged Care: Enhanced version May 2006.* Canberra: Australian Government Department of Health and Ageing.

Conway, M.A., Wang, Q., Hanyu, K. and Haque, S. (2005) 'A Cross-Cultural Investigation of Autobiographical Memory.' *Journal of Cross-Cultural Psychology 36,* 6, 739–49.

Cooke, G. (2001) *Being with God.* Sydney: Dayspring Direct.

Crowther, M.R., Parker, M.R., Achenbaum, W.A., Larimore, W.L. and Koenig, H.G. (2002) 'Rowe and Kahn's Model of Successful Ageing Revisited: Positive Spirituality – the Forgotten Factor.' *The Gerontologist 42,* 5, 613–20.

Daaleman, T., and Frey, B. (2004) 'The Spirituality Index of Well-Being: A New Instrument for Health-Related Quality-of-Life Research.' *Annals of Family Medicine 2*, 5.

Damasio, A. (2003) *Looking for Spinoza: Joy, Sorrow and the Feeling Brain.* Orlando, FL: Harcourt Inc.

Davis, L. (2005) 'Educating Individuals with Dementia.' *Topics in Geriatric Rehabilitation 21*, 4, 304–14.

Davison, E.H., Pless, A.P., Gugliucci, M.R., King, L.A., King, D.W., Salgado, D.M., Spiro, A. and Bachrach, P. (2006) 'Late-Life Emergence of Early-Life Trauma: The Phenomenon of Late-Onset Stress Symptomatology among Aging Combat Veterans.' *Research on Aging 28*, 1, 84–114.

Dayal, H. (1932) *The Bodhisattva Doctrine in Buddhist Sanskrit Literature.* Delhi: Motilal Banarsidass.

de Grucy, J. (ed.) (1996) *The Cambridge Companion to Dietrich Bonhoeffer.* Cambridge: Cambridge University Press.

De Leo, D. (2002) 'Struggling against suicide: The Need for an Integrative Approach.' *Crisis: The Journal of Crisis Intervention and Suicide Prevention 23*, 1, 23–31.

De Leo, D., Hickey, P.A., Neulinger, K. and Cantor, C.H. (2001) *Ageing and Suicide.* Canberra: Commonwealth of Australia.

Derrida, J. (1976) *Of Grammatology*, trans. G.C. Spivak. Baltimore, MD: The John Hopkins University Press.

Dictionary.com Unabridged (n.d.) 'Blessing.' Random House, Inc. Accessed on 5 February 2005 at: http://dictionary.reference.com/browse/blessing

Diener, E. and Clifton, D. (2002) 'Life Satisfaction and Religiosity in Broad Probability Samples.' *Psychological Inquiry 13*, 3, 206–9.

Doogue, G. and Sturgess, W. (2005) *Happiness.* Sydney: ABC.

Driver, T. (1991) *The Magic of Ritual.* San Francisco, CA: Harper Collins.

Dudley, M. and Koder, S. (2002) 'Religion, Spirituality and Psychiatry: A Review Essay.' *Uniting Church Studies 8*, 1, 14–41.

Eiesland, N.L. (1994) *The Disabled God: Toward a Liberatory Theology of Disability.* Nashville, TN: Abingdon Press.

Eisenhandler, S.A. (1999) 'Reading between the Lines: Aspects of Transcendence and Spirituality in One Group.' In L.E. Thomas and S.A. Eisenhandler (eds) *Religion, Belief, and Spirituality in Late Life.* New York, NY: Springer.

Ellison, C.G. (1994) 'Religion, the Life Stress Paradigm, and the Study of Depression.' In J.S. Levin (ed.) *Religion in Aging and Health.* Thousand Oaks, CA: Sage.

Engelhardt, H.T. (1986) *The Foundations of Bioethics.* New York, NY: Oxford University Press.

Erikson, E. (1963) *Childhood and Society* (2nd edn). New York, NY: Norton.

Erikson, E., Erikson, J and Kivnick, H. (1986) *Vital Involvement in Old Age: The Experience of Old Age in Our Time.* New York, NY: Norton.

Evans, B.J., Burrows, G.D. and Norman, T.R. (2000) *Understanding Depression.* Melbourne: Mental Health Promotion Unit, University of Melbourne.

Federation of L'Arche (1993) 'The Charter of the Communities of L'Arche', Resources: Official Documents. Accessed on 6 April 2007 at: www.larche.org

Feenstra, R.J., and Plantinga, C. (1989) *Trinity, Incarnation and Atonement: Philosophical and Theological Essays.* University of Notre Dame, IN: Notre Dame Press.

Flannery, A. (ed.) (1977) *Vatican II. The Conciliar and Post Conciliar Documents.* Dublin: Dominican Publications.

Fleming, R. (2001a) *Challenge Depression.* Canberra: Commonwealth Department of Health and Ageing.

Fleming, R. (2001b) 'Depression and Spirituality in Australian Aged Care Homes.' *Journal of Religious Gerontology, 13,* 3/ 4, 107–16.

Fleming, R. (2004) *Challenging Depression in the Elderly: Making a Determined Start* (Discussion paper). Sydney: The Hammond Care Group.

Folstein, M., Folstein, S. and McHugh, P. (1975) 'Mini-Mental State: A Practical Method for Grading the Cognitive State of Patients for the Clinician.' *Journal of Psychiatry Research 12,* 185–98.

Fowler, J.W. (1981) *Stages of Faith: The Psychology of Human Development and the Quest for Meaning.* San Francisco, CA: Harper.

Fowler, J.W. (2004) 'Faith Development at 30: Naming the Challenges of Faith in a New Millennium.' *Religious Education 99,* 4, 405–21.

Frankl, V.E. (1984) *Man's Search for Meaning.* New York, NY: Washington Square Press.

Freedman, D.N. (ed.) (1992) *The Anchor Bible Dictionary.* New York, NY: Doubleday.

French, B.M. (1995) 'Dementia.' *The University of Alberta's Cognitive Science Dictionary.* Accessed on 8 August 2007 at: http://penta.ufrgs.br/edu/telelab/3/dementia.htm

French, S. and Swain, J. (2002) 'Across the Disability Divide: Whose Tragedy?' In K.W.M. Fulford, D.L. Dickenson and T.H. Murray (eds) *Healthcare Ethics and Human Values: An Introductory Text with Readings and Case Studies.* Oxford: Blackwell.

Frey, B., Daaleman, T. and Peyton, V. (2005) 'Measuring a Dimension of Spirituality for Health Research: Validity of the Spirituality Index of Well-Being.' *Research On Aging 27,* 5, 556–77.

Friedman, D. (2003) 'An Anchor amidst Anomie: Ritual and Aging.' In M. Kimble and S. McFadden (eds) *Aging, Spirituality and Religion: A Handbook, Volume 2.* Minneapolis, MN: Fortress.

Fulghum, R. (1995) *From Beginning to End: The Rituals of our Lives.* New York, NY: Random House.

Gardner, W.L., Pickett, C.L. and Brewer, M.B. (2000) 'Social Exclusion and Selective Memory: How the Need to Belong Influences Memory for Social Events.' *Personality and Social Psychology Bulletin 26*, 4, 486–96.

Gennep, A. van (1909/1960) *The Rites of Passage*, trans. M. Vizedom and G. Caffee. Chicago, IL: University of Chicago Press.

George, L.K., Hays, J.C., Flint, E.P. and Meador, K.G. (2004) 'Religion and Health in Life Course Perspective.' In K.W. Schaie, N.M. Krause and A. Booth (eds) *Religious Influences on Health and Well-Being in the Elderly.* New York, NY: Springer.

Gerkin, C.V. (1984) *The Living Human Document: Re-Visioning Pastoral Counselling in a Hermeneutical Mode.* Nashville, TN: Abingdon.

Gerster, R. (1987) *Big-Noting: The Heroic Theme in Australian War Writing.* Carlton: Melbourne University Press.

Gibson, F. (1998) *Reminiscence and Recall: A Guide to Good Practice* (2nd edn). Devon: Age Concern Books.

Gibson, G. and Gibson, R. (1991) *The Sandwich Generation.* Grand Rapids, MI: Baker Book House.

Glaser, B.G. and Strauss, A. (1967) *The Discovery of Grounded Theory: Strategies for Qualitative Research.* New York, NY: Aldine de Gruyter.

Goggin, G. and Newell, C. (2004) 'Uniting the Nation?: Disability, Stem Cells, and the Australian Media.' *Disability & Society 19*, 1, January, 47–60.

Goggin, G. and Newell, C. (2005) *Disability in Australia: Exposing a Social Apartheid.* Sydney: UNSW Press.

Goldberg, M. (1991) *Theology and Narrative: A Critical Introduction.* Philadelphia, PA: Trinity Press International.

Goldsmith, M. (2004) *In a Strange Land: People with Dementia and the Local Church.* Southwell: 4M Publications.

Goldsmith, M. (2007) Unpublished work in progress.

Goulart, J. (2005) *God Has No Religion: Blending Traditions for Prayer.* Notre Dame, IN: Sorin Books.

Habermas, J. (1981) *Communication and the Evolution of Society.* Boston, MA: Beacon Press.

Haight, B.K. and Webster, J.D. (eds) (1995) *The Art and Science of Reminiscing: Theory, Research, Methods, and Applications.* Washington, DC: Taylor and Francis.

Hales, C., Ross, L. and Ryan, C. (2006) 'National Evaluation of the Aged Care Innovative Pool Dementia Pilot: Final Report.' Canberra: Australian Institute of Health and Welfare. Accessed on 15 March 2007 at: www.aihw.gov.au/publications/age/neacipdp/neacipdp.pdf

Hall, K. (2006) Letter to the author.

Hallahan, L. (2005) *In My Flesh Shall I See God: Journeys Through Disability and Theology.* Unpublished Doctoral Thesis: Flinders University.

Halpern, A. (1988) 'Perceived and Imagined Tempos of Familiar Songs.' *Memory and Perception 6*, 193–202.

Halpern, A. (1989) 'Memory for the Absolute Pitch of Familiar Songs.' *Memory and Cognition 17*, 5, 572–81.

Hauerwas, S. (1986). *Suffering Presence: Theological Reflections on Medicine, the Mentally Handicapped, and the Church.* Notre Dame, IN: University of Notre Dame Press.

Hauerwas, S. (2004a) 'Timeful Friends: Living with the Handicapped.' In J. Swinton (ed.) *Critical Reflections on Stanley Hauerwas' Theology of Disability: Disabling Society, Enabling Theology.* New York, NY: Haworth Pastoral Press, 11–26.

Hauerwas, S. (2004b) 'Reflection on Dependency: A Response to Responses to My Essays on Disability.' In J. Swinton (ed.) *Critical Reflections on Stanley Hauerwas' Theology of Disability: Disabling Society, Enabling Theology.* New York, NY: Haworth Pastoral Press, 191–8.

Hauerwas, S. and Jones, L.G. (eds) (1989) *Why Narrative?* Grand Rapids, MI: Eerdmans.

Hauerwas, S., Stoneking, C.B., Meador, K.G. and Cloutier, D. (eds) (2003) *Growing Old in Christ.* Grand Rapids, MI: Eerdmans.

Herr, S. and Weber, G. (eds) (1999) *Aging, Rights, and Quality of Life: Prospects for Older People with Developmental Disabilities.* Baltimore, MD: Paul H. Brookes Publishing Co.

Hickie, I.B., Simons, L., Naismith, S., Simons, J., McCallum, J. and Pearson, K. (2003) 'Vascular Risk to Late-Life Depression: Evidence from a Longitudinal Community Study.' *Australian and New Zealand Journal of Psychiatry 37*, 1, 62–5.

Hill, R.D., Gallagher, D., Thompson, H.W. and Ishida, T. (1998) 'Hopelessness as a Measure of Suicidal Intent in the Depressed Elderly.' *Psychology and Aging 3*, 3, 230–2.

Hudson, R. (2004a) 'Ageing and the Trinity: Holey, Wholly, Holy?' In A. Jewell (ed.) *Ageing, Spirituality and Well-Being.* London: Jessica Kingsley Publishers, 86–100.

Hudson, R. (2004b) 'Dementia and Personhood: A Living Death or Alive in God? Colloquium.' *The Australian and New Zealand Theological Review 36*, 2, 123–42.

Huggett, J. (1988) *Formed by the Desert.* Guildford: Eagle.

Hughes, J.C., Louw, S.J. and Sabat S.R. (eds) (2006). *Dementia, Mind, Meaning, and the Person.* Oxford: Oxford University Press.

Hutchison, M.G. (1997) 'Unity and Diversity in Spiritual Care.' Paper originally presented at the Sydney University Nursing Society First Annual Conference for Undergraduate Nursing Students in NSW, September.

Idler, E.L. (2004) 'Religious Observance and Health: Theory and Research.' In K.W. Schaie, N.M. Krause and A. Booth (eds) *Religious Influences on Health and Well-Being in the Elderly.* New York, NY: Springer.

Imber-Black, E., and Roberts, J. (1992) *Rituals for our Time: Celebrating, Healing and Changing Our Lives and Our Relationships.* New York, NY: Harper Collins.

Iozzio, M.J. (2005) 'The Writing on the Wall…Alzheimer's Disease A Daughter's Look at Mom's Faithful Care of Dad.' *Journal of Religion, Disability and Health 9*, 2, 49–80. New York, NY: Haworth Press.

Isaiah, D., Parker, V. and Murrow, E. (1999) 'Spiritual Well-Being among Older Adults.' *Journal of Gerontology 25*, 8, 15–21.

Jackson, J.P. (2006a) 'Isolation: A Subtle Deception.' *The Morning Star Journal, 16*, 1, 45–9.

Jackson, J.P. (2006b) *Seven Days Behind the Veil: Throne Room Meditations.* North Sutton, NH: Streams Publishing House.

Jamieson, D. (2005) *Exploring and Affirming My Life: A Short Course in Spiritual Reminiscence Work* (2nd edn). Canberra: Centre for Ageing & Pastoral Studies.

Jayatilake, K.N. (1963) *Early Buddhist Theory of Knowledge.* London: George Allen and Unwin Ltd.

Jeremiah, M. (2003) *Alone with Dementia.* Published privately, obtainable from 43 Boat Dyke Road, Upton, Norwich.

Jewell, A. (ed) (1999) *Spirituality and Ageing.* London: Jessica Kingsley Publishers.

Jewell, A. (ed) (2004) *Ageing, Spirituality and Well-Being.* London: Jessica Kingsley Publishers.

Johnson, J. and Ulatowska, H. (1996) 'The Nature of Tune and Text in the Production of songs.' In R. Pratt and R. Spingte (eds) *Music and Medicine 2.* St Louis, MO: MMB Music, 153–69.

Johnston, M. (2002) *At the Front Line.* Cambridge: Cambridge University Press.

Jones, T.P. (2004) 'The Basis of James W. Fowler's Understanding of Faith in the Research of Wilfred Cantwell Smith: An Examination from an Evangelical Perspective.' *Religious Education 99*, 4, 1–8.

Jorm, A.F., Griffiths, K.M., Christensen, H., Parslow, R.A. and Rodgers, B. (2004) 'Actions Taken to Cope with Depression at Different Levels of Severity: A Community Survey.' *Psychological Medicine, 34*, 293–9.

Joyner, R. (2005a) *The Fruit of the Land, part IV.* Accessed on 30 July 2005 at: http://morningstarministries.org/pages/word_week/2005/3005.htm

Joyner, R. (2005b) *The Fruit of the Land, part VII.* Accessed on 7 August 2005 at: http://morningstarministries.org/pages/word_week/2005/3105.htm

Joyner, R. (2005c) *Taking the Land, part V.* Accessed on 13 December 2005 at: http://morningstarministries.org/pages/word_week/2005/3105.htm

Kaldor, P., Bellamy, J. and Powell, R. (1997) *Shaping a Future: Characteristics of Vital Congregations.* Adelaide: Openbook.

Kaldor, P., Dixon, R. and Powell, R. (1999) *Taking Stock: A Profile of Australian Church Attenders.* Adelaide: Openbook.

Kalupahana, D.J. (1976) *Buddhist Philosophy: A Historical Analysis.* Honolulu: The University Press of Hawaii.

Kaplan, H.I. and Sadock, B.J. (1991) *Synopsis of Psychiatry.* Baltimore, MA: Williams and Wilkins.

Kass, L.R. (2003) *The Beginning of Wisdom: Reading Genesis.* New York, NY: Free Press.

Kaszniak, A. and Christenson, G. (1994) 'Differential Diagnosis of Dementia and Depression.' In M. Storandt and G. VandenBos (eds) *Neuropsychological Assessment of Dementia and Depression in Older Adults: A Clinician's Guide.* Washington, DC: American Psychological Society.

Katz, S. and Marshall, B. (2003) 'New Sex for Old: Lifestyle, Consumerism, and the Ethics of Aging Well.' *Journal of Aging Studies 17,* 3–16.

Kaut, K. (2002) 'Religion, Spirituality and Existentialism Near the End of Life.' *American Behavioural Scientist 46,* 220–34.

Kehn, D.J. (1995) 'Predictors of Elderly Happiness.' *Activities, Adaptation and Aging 19,* 3, 11–30.

Kelly, A. (1989) *The Trinity of Love: A Theology of the Christian God.* Wilmington, DE: Michael Glazier Wilmington.

Kelly, K. (2006) Letter to the author.

Kenyon, G.M., Clark, P. and de Vries, B. (2001) (eds) *Narrative Gerontology: Theory, Research, and Practice.* New York, NY: Springer.

Killick, J. (2006) 'Helping the Flame to Stay Bright: Celebrating the Spiritual in Dementia.' *Journal of Religion, Spirituality and Aging 18,* 2/3, 73–8.

Killick, J. and Allan, K. (2001) *Communication and the Care of People with Dementia.* Buckingham: Open University Press.

Kimble, M.A. (1990) 'Aging and the Search for Meaning.' In Seeber, J.J. (ed.) *Spiritual Maturity in the Later Years.* New York, NY: Haworth Pastoral Press.

Kimble, M.A. (2001) 'A Personal Journey of Aging: The Spiritual Dimension.' In S.H McFadden and R.C. Atchley (eds) *Aging and the Meaning of Time: A Multidisciplinary Exploration.* New York, NY: Springer Publishing Company.

Kimble, M.A. (2003) 'Final Time: Coming to the End.' In M.A. Kimble and S.H. McFadden (eds) *Aging, Spirituality and Religion: A Handbook, Volume 2.* Minneapolis, MN: Fortress Press.

Kitwood, T. (1995) 'Toward the Reconstruction of an Organic Mental Disorder.' In A. Radley (ed.) *Worlds of Illness: Biographical and Cultural Perspectives on Health and Disease.* London: Routledge.

Kitwood, T. (1997) *Dementia Reconsidered.* Buckingham: Open University Press.

Knox, I.S. (2002) *Older People and the Church.* Edinburgh: T. & T. Clark.

Koenig, H.G. (1994) *Aging and God: Spiritual Pathways to Mental Health in Midlife and Later Years.* New York, NY: The Haworth Pastoral Press.

Koenig, H.G. (ed) (1998) *Handbook of Religion and Mental Health.* San Diego, CA: Academic Press.

Koenig, H.G. and Kuchibhatia, M. (1999) 'Use of Health Services by Medically Ill Depressed Elderly Patients after Hospital Discharge.' *American Journal of Geriatric Psychiatry 7,* 48–56.

Koenig, H.G. and Weaver, A.J. (1998) *Pastoral Care of Older Adults: Creative Pastoral Care and Counselling.* Minneapolis, MN: Fortress Press.

Koenig, H.G., Cohen, H.J., George, L.K. *et al.* (1997) 'Attendance at Religious Services, Interleukin-6, and Other Biological Parameters of Immune Function in Older Adults.' *International Journal of Psychiatry in Medicine 27*, 3, 233–50.

Koenig, H.G., McCullough, M. and Larson, D. (2001) *Handbook of Religion and Health.* New York, NY: Oxford University Press.

Kopelman, L.M. (1996) 'Ethical Assumptions and Ambiguities in the Americans with Disabilities Act.' *Journal of Medicine and Philosophy 21*, 194.

Krause, N.M. (2003) 'Religious Meaning and Subjective Well-Being in Late Life.' *The Journals of Gerontology: Series B: Psychological and Social Sciences 58B*, 3, S160 cf.

Kugel, J.L. (2003) *The God of Old: Inside the Lost World of the Bible.* New York, NY: The Free Press.

L'Arche Ontario (2005) Vison Statement: Ageing, Grieving & Dying: Internal Resources. Accessed on 6 April 2007 at: www.larche.ca/en/members/aging

LaCugna, C. (1991). *God for Us: The Trinity and Christian Life.* San Francisco, CA: Harper.

Laffin, J. (1959) *Digger: The Story of the Australian Soldier.* London: Cassell.

Lake-Smith, T. (2006) Personal communication.

Lambert, E. (1952) *The Twenty Thousand Thieves.* London: Muller.

Lapsley, J. (1969) 'Pastoral Theology Past and Present.' In W.B. Oglesby Jr. (ed.) *The New Shape of Pastoral Theology: Essays in Honor of Seward Hiltner.* Nashville, TN: Abingdon Press.

Laugesen, A. (2003) 'Australian First World War "Slanguage".' *Journal of the Australian War Memorial 38*, April. Accessed on 11 December 2006 at: www.awm.gov.au/journal/j38/ slanguage.htm

Law, B.C. (1986) *Concepts of Buddhism.* Delhi: Gian Publishing House.

Lear, J. (1988) *Aristotle: The Desire to Understand.* Cambridge: Cambridge University Press.

Lee, J. (1994) *The Empowerment Approach to Social Work Practice.* New York, NY: Columbia University Press.

Lefcourt, H. (2001) *The Psychology of Living Buoyantly.* New York, NY: Plenum.

Levin, J.S. and Taylor, R.J. (1997) 'Age Differences in Patterns and Correlates of the Frequency of Prayer.' *The Gerontologist 37*, 1, 75–88.

Lewis, A. (1982) 'God as Cripple: Disability, Personhood and the Reign of God.' *Pacific Theological Review 16*, 1, 13–18.

Lewis, J. (1996) *The Monkey Rope: A Psychotherapist's Reflections on Relationships.* New York, NY: Bernel.

Llewellyn-Jones, R. (2004) 'New Approaches for Late Life Depression.' *Proceedings of the Maturity Blues Conference, Powerhouse Museum, Sydney (Australia), 24 June 2004.* Accessed on 8 June 2005 at: www.beyondblue.org.au

Looi, Jeffrey. (2005) *Depression goes unnoticed among elderly.* Jan 17 report, ABC Newsonline. Sydney: ABC.

Lunsford, D.A. and Burnett, M.S. (1992) 'Marketing Product Innovations to the Elderly: Understanding the Barriers to Adoption.' *Journal of Consumer Marketing 9*, 53–64.

McBee, L. (2003) 'Mindfulness Practice with the Frail Elderly and Their Caregivers in Topics.' *Geriatric Rehabilitation 19*, 4, 257–64.

McFadden, S.H. (1996) 'Religion, Spirituality, and Aging.' In J.E. Birren and K.W. Schaie (eds) *Handbook of the Psychology of Aging.* San Diego, CA: Academic Press.

McFadden, S.H. (2004) 'The Paradoxes of Humour and the Burden of Despair.' In E. MacKinley (ed.) *Spirituality of Later Life: On Humor and Despair.* New York, NY: Haworth Pastoral Press.

MacIntyre, A. (1999) *Dependent Rational Animals: Why Human Beings Need the Virtues.* Chicago, IL: Open Court.

McKee, K.J., Wilson, F., Chung, M.C. *et al.* (2005) 'Reminiscence, Regrets and Activity in Older People in Residential Health Care: Associations with Psychological Health.' *British Journal of Clinical Psychology 44*, 534–61.

MacKinlay, E. (1998) *The Spiritual Dimension of Ageing: Meaning in Life, Response to Meaning, and Well Being in Ageing* (doctoral thesis). Melbourne: La Trobe University.

MacKinlay, E. (2001a) *The Spiritual Dimension of Ageing.* London: Jessica Kingsley Publishers.

MacKinlay, E. (2001b) 'The Spiritual Dimension of Caring: Applying a Model for Spiritual Tasks of Ageing.' *Journal of Religious Gerontology 12*, 3/4, 151–66.

MacKinlay, E. (2002) 'Mental Health and Spirituality in Later Life: Pastoral Approaches.' *Journal of Religious Gerontology 13*, 3/4, 129–47.

MacKinlay E. (2004) 'Humour: A Way to Transcendence in Later Life?' In E. MacKinlay (ed.) *Spirituality of Later Life: On Humor and Despair.* New York, NY: Haworth Pastoral Press.

MacKinlay, E. (2006a) *Spiritual Growth and Care in the Fourth Age of Life.* London: Jessica Kingsley Publishers.

MacKinlay, E. (ed.) (2006b) *Aging, Spirituality and Palliative Care.* New York, NY: Haworth Press.

MacKinlay, E. and Trevitt, C. (2006) *Facilitating Spiritual Reminiscence for Older People with Dementia: A Learning Package.* Canberra: CAPS Publishing.

MacKinlay, E., Ellor, J.W. and Pickard, S. (eds) (2001) *Aging, Spirituality and Pastoral Care: A Multi-National Perspective.* New York, NY: The Haworth Pastoral Press.

MacKinlay, E., Trevitt, C. and Coady, M. (2002–2005) *Finding Meaning in the Experience of Dementia: The Place of Spiritual Reminiscence Work.* Unpublished research project. Australian Research Council, Linkage Grant 2002–2005.

Macleod, D. (2005) *Fowler Faith Development.* Accessed on 19 July 2006 at: http://www.generations.postkiwi.com

McSherry, W. (2006) *Making Sense of Spirituality in Nursing and Health Care Practice.* London: Jessica Kingsley Publishers.

Maddox, G.L. (2001) 'Disability.' In G.L. Maddox (ed.) *The Encyclopedia of Aging.* New York, NY: Springer.

Magalhães, João Pedro (2005) *What Is Ageing?* Accessed on 15 March 2007 at: www.senescence.info/definitions.html

Martin, R.A. (1998) 'Approaches to the Sense of Humor: A Historical Review.' In W. Ruch (ed.) *The Sense of Humor: Explorations of a Personality Characteristic.* Berlin: Mouton de Gruyter.

Mauritzen, J. (1988) 'Pastoral Care for the Dying and Bereaved.' *Death Studies 12,* 111–12 [Cited in Kaut 2002].

May, W.F. (1986) 'The Virtues and Vices of the Elderly.' In T.R. Cole and S.A. Gadow (eds) *What Does It Mean to Grow Old?* Durham: Duke University Press.

Meador, K.G. (2004) 'Spiritual Care at the End of Life.' *North Carolina Medical Journal 65,* 4, 226–8.

Meares, R. (2000) *Intimacy and Alienation: Memory, Trauma and Personal Being.* London: Routledge.

Meares, R. (2005) 'Analogical Structure of the Narrative of Self.' In R. Meares and P. Nolan (eds) *The Self in Conversation.* Sydney: ANZAP.

Meilaender, G. (1991). 'I Want to Burden My Loved Ones.' *First Things,* 16 October, 12–16.

Mitchell, J. (1989) 'Pastoral Care and Ritual.' *Journal of Pastoral Care 43,* 68–77.

Moberg, D.O. (ed.) (2001) *Aging and Spirituality: Spiritual Dimensions of Aging Theory, Research, Practice, and Policy.* New York, NY: The Haworth Pastoral Press.

Moberg, D.O. (2005) 'Research in Spirituality, Religion, and Aging.' *Journal of Gerontological Social Work 45,* 1/ 2, 11–40.

Moltmann, J. (1977) *The Church in the Power of the Spirit.* London: SCM.

Moltmann, J. (1985) *God in Creation: An Ecological Doctrine of Creation.* London: SCM Press Ltd.

Moltmann, J. (1993) *The Trinity and the Kingdom of God: The Doctrine of God.* London: SCM Press Ltd.

Moody, H.R. (2005) *Religion, Spirituality and Aging: A Social Work Perspective.* Binghamton, NY: The Haworth Social Work Practice Press.

Moore, H. (1994) *A Passion for Difference.* Cambridge: Polity Press.

Moran, C. (2003) 'Beyond Content: Does Humor Use Help Coping?' *Disability Studies Quarterly 3,* 1–5 (e-journal).

Moran, C. (2004) 'Allies Cartoon Humor in World War II: A Comparison of Willie and Joe and Bluey and Curley.' *International Journal of Comic Art 6,* 2, 431–44.

Moran, C. (2005) 'Humour and Meaning after Trauma.' *Psychology, Psychiatry, and Mental Health Monographs: Trauma: Responses Across the Lifespan* (Parramatta: NSWIOP) 2, Nov, 113–24.

Moran, C. and Massam, M. (2003) 'A "Trace of History": Cartoons from the Australian War Memorial Christmas Books of the Second World War.' *Journal of the Australian War Memorial v39,* October 2003. Accessed on 11 December 2006 at: www.awm.gov.au/journal/j39/cartoons.htm

Morgan, R.L. (1995) 'Guiding Spiritual Autobiography for Third and Fourth Agers.' *Journal of Religious Gerontology 9,* 2, 1–14.

Moriarty, G. (2006) *Pastoral Care of Depression.* New York, NY: Haworth Press.

Morley, J. (1992) *All Desires Known.* London: SPCK.

Nakamura, J. and Csikszentmihalyi, M. (2003) 'Creativity in Later Life.' In R. Sawyer and V. John-Steiner (eds) *Creativity and Development.* New York, NY: Oxford University Press.

Nānamoli (Tr) (1979) *Path of Purification* (3rd edn). Kandy, Sri Lanka: Buddhist Publication Society.

National Institute of Mental Health Press Office (2005) *Cognitive Therapy Reduces Repeat Suicide Attempts by 50 percent.* Press release, Canberra: NIMH.

Nelson, H.L. (2001) *Damaged Identities, Narrative Repair.* Ithaca, NY: Cornell University Press.

Newell, C. (1996) 'Critical Reflections on Euthanasia and People with Disability.' *Australian Quarterly 68,* 3, Spring, 48–56.

Newell, C. (2000) 'Euthanasia, Disability and Christian Ethics: A Clash of Cultures?' In M. Free *et al.* (eds) *That Our Joy May Be Complete: Essays on the Incarnation for the New Millennium.* Adelaide: Openbook Publishers, 97–111.

Newell, C. (2006) 'Love and Healing.' *Dialogue Australasia 15,* April, 3–5.

Newell, C. and Calder, A. (eds) (2004) *Voices in Spirituality and Disability from the Land Down Under: From Out Back to Out Front.* Birmingham, NY: Haworth Press.

Noon, B. (2003) 'Burning Bright.' In S. Benson and J. Killick *Creativity in Dementia Care Calendar 2004.* London: Hawker.

Northcott, M. (1993) 'New Age Rites: The Recovery of Ritual.' *The Way 33,* 3, 189–98.

Nouwen, H.J.M. (1972) *The Wounded Healer: Ministry in Contemporary Society.* Garden City, NY: Doubleday.

Nyanatiloka (1980) *Buddhist Dictionary: Manual of Buddhist Terms and Doctrines.* Kandy, Sri Lanka: Buddhist Publication Society.

O'Connor, D.W., Rosewarne, R. and Bruce, A. (2001) 'Depression in Primary Care 1: Elderly Patients' Disclosure of Depressive Symptoms to Their Doctors.' *International Psychogeriatrics 13,* 3, 359–65.

Paige, A. (1994) *Coming Apart, Coming Together: One Man's Journey Out of Depression.* Liguori, MO: Liguori Publications.

Palapathwala, R. (2006a) *Cosmogonic Myths as Pathways to Interfaith Dialogue.* Kerala, Karickam: Dr Alexander Marthom Centre for Dialogue.

Palapathwala, R. (2006b) 'Ageing and Death: A Buddhist-Christian Conceptual Framework for Spirituality in Later Life.' In E. MacKinlay (ed.) *Aging, Spirituality and Palliative Care.* Binghamton, NY: The Haworth Pastoral Press, 153–68.

Pali Text Society (ed.) (1913) *Sutta Nipatta.*

Pali Text Society (ed.) (1884–1904) *Samyutta Nikāyā.*

Palmer, P.J. (2004) *A Hidden Wholeness: The Journey toward an Undivided Life. Welcoming the Soul and Weaving Community in a Wounded World.* San Francisco, CA: Jossey-Bass.

Papalia, D.E. and Olds, S.W. (1992) *Human Development* (5th edn). New York, NY: McGraw-Hill.

Pargament, K.I. and Ano, G.G. (2004) 'Empirical Advances in the Psychology of Religion and Coping.' In K.W. Schaie, N.M. Krause and A. Booth (eds) *Religious Influences on Health and Well-Being in the Elderly.* New York, NY: Springer.

Parliament of Australia Library (2002) *Disability Support and Services in Australia.* Accessed on 15 March 2007 at: www.aph.gov.au/library/intguide/sp/disability.htm

Peach, H.G. (2003) 'Religion, Spirituality and Health: How should Australia's Medical Professionals Respond?' *Medical Journal of Australia 178,* 2, 86–8.

Peretz, I., Gagnon, L., Hébert, S. and Macoir, J. (2004) 'Singing in the Brain: Insights from Cognitive Neuropsychology.' *Music Perception 21,* 3, 373–90.

Perlmutter, M. (1988) 'Cognitive Potential Throughout Life.' In H. Birren and V. Bengtson (eds) *Emergent Theories of Aging.* New York, NY: Springer, 247–68.

Piolino, P., Desgranges, B., Clarys, D. *et al.* (2006) 'Autobiographical Memory, Autonoetic Consciousness, and Self-Perspective in Aging.' *Psychology and Aging 21,* 3, 510–25.

Pontifical Council for Justice and Peace (2005) *Compendium of the Social Doctrine of the Church.* Strathfield: St Pauls.

Post, S.G. (1995) *The Moral Challenge of Alzheimer Disease.* Baltimore: The Johns Hopkins University Press.

Post, S.G. (2000) *The Moral Challenge of Alzheimer Disease* (2nd edn). Baltimore, MD: The Johns Hopkins University Press.

Proctor-Smith, M. (1990) *In Her Own Rite: Constructing Feminist Liturgical Tradition.* Nashville, TN: Abingdon.

Rabins, P., Kasper, J., Kleinman, L., Black, B. and Patrick, D. (1999) 'Concepts and Methods in the Development of the ADRQL: An Instrument for Assessing Heath-Related Quality of Life in Persons with Alzheimer's Disease.' *Journal of Mental Health and Aging 5,* 33–48.

Ramshaw, E. (1987) *Ritual and Pastoral Care.* Philadelphia, PA: Fortress.

Rappaport, J. (1981) 'In Praise of Paradox: A Social Policy of Empowerment over Prevention.' *American Journal of Community Psychology 9,*1, 1–25.

Reinders, H.S. (2000) *The Future of the Disabled in Liberal Society: An Ethical Analysis.* Notre Dame, ID: University of Notre Dame Press.

Renner, P. (1979) 'The Use of Ritual in Pastoral Care.' *Journal of Pastoral Care 23,* 165–6.

Rich, A. (1981) 'The Spirit of Place.' In A. Rich, *A Wild Patience Has Taken Me this Far: Poems 1978–1981.* New York, NY: W.W. Norton.

Richards, T. (2002) *NVivo 2*. Australia: QSR International.

Ricoeur, P. (2004) *Memory, History, Forgetting*, trans. by K. Blamey and D. Pellauer. Chicago, IL: University of Chicago Press.

Robertson-Gillam, K. (1995) 'Music Therapy Can Meet the Spiritual Needs of Dying People.' In C. Lee (ed.) *Lonely Waters*. Oxford, England: Michael Sobell House.

Rost, R.A. (2005) 'Spiritual Need Five: Providing Quality Pastoral Care as a Congregation.' In D.R. Koepke (ed.) *Ministering to Older Adults: The Building Blocks*. New York, NY: The Haworth Pastoral Press.

Rowe, J. and Kahn, R. (1997) 'Successful Aging.' *The Gerontologist 37*, 433–440.

Ruch, W. (ed.) (1998) *The Sense of Humor: Explorations of a Personality Characteristic*. Berlin: Mouton de Gruyter.

Rudin, M. (2006) *The Science of Happiness*. Accessed on 8 May 2006 at: http://newsvote.bbc.co.uk

Rudman, S. (1997) *Concepts of Persons and Christian Ethics*. London: Cambridge University Press.

Ruzich, M.J., Looi, J.C.L. and Robertson, M.D. (2005) 'Delayed Onset Posttraumic Stress Disorder among Male Combat Veterans.' *American Geriatric Psychiatry 13*, 5, 425–7.

Sacks, O. (1985) *The Man who Mistook his Wife for a Hat and Other Clinical Tales*. New York, NY: Harper and Row.

Sarna, N.M. (1989) *The JPS Torah Commentary: Genesis*. Philadelphia, PA: Jewish Publication Society.

Schnurr, P.P. (1991) 'PTSD and Combat-Related Psychiatric Symptoms in Older Veterans.' *PTSD Research Quarterly 2*, 1, 1–8.

Scobie, C. (2006) 'Songs to Remember.' *Sun-Herald*, 8 October, Sunday Life magazine, 25–27 (Sydney, Australia: Fairfax Newspapers).

Scott, C. (2006) Circular Letter.

Scott-Holland, H. (1910) Words from a sermon preached in St Paul's Cathedral whilst the body of king Edward VII was laying in state at Westminster. Published in *Facts of the Faith* in 1919.

Scott-Maxwell, F. (1968) *The Measure of My Days*. New York, NY: Alfred Knopf.

Senior, D. (1995) 'Beware of the Canaanite Woman: Disability and the Bible.' In M.E. Bishop (ed.) *Religion and Disability*. Kansas City, KS: Sheed and Ward.

Shammi, P. and Stuss, D.T. (2003) 'The effects of Normal Aging on Humor Appreciation.' *Journal of the International Neuropsychological Society 9*, 6 855–63.

Shamy, E. (1997) *More than Body, Brain and Breath*. Re-published in England in 2003 as *A Guide to the Spiritual Dimension of Care for People with Alzheimer's Disease and Related Dementia*. London: Jessica Kingsley Publishers.

Shulik, R.N. (1992) 'Faith Development in Older Adults.' In J. Astley and L.J. Francis (eds) *Christian Perspectives on Faith Development*. Leominster: Gracewing.

Silvers, A. (1996) '(In)equality, (ab)normality, and the Americans with Disabilities Act.' *Journal of Medicine and Philosophy 21*, 211–12.

Singer, P. (1993) *Practical Ethics* (2nd edn). Cambridge: Cambridge University Press.

Sixsmith, A. Stilwell, J. and Copeland, J. (1993) '"Rementia": Challenging the limits of dementia care.' *International Journal of Geriatric Psychiatry 8*, 12, 993–1000.

Snudden, P. (2006) Letter to the author.

Snyder, C and Lopez, S. (eds) (2002) *Handbook of Positive Psychology*. New York, NY: Oxford University Press.

Snyder, C.R., Sigmon, D.R. and Feldman, D.B. (2002) 'Hope for the Sacred and Vice Versa: Positive Goal-Directed Thinking and Religion.' *Psychological Inquiry 13*, 3, 234–8.

Sorrell, J. (2006) 'Listening in Thin Places: Ethics in the Care of Persons with Alzheimer's Disease.' *Advances in Nursing Science 29*, 2, 152–61.

Sperry, L. (1992) 'Aging: A Developmental Perspective.' *Individual Psychology 48*, 4.

Sprod, G. (1981) *Bamboo Round My Shoulder: Changi, the Lighter Side.* Kenthurst, NSW: Kangaroo Press.

Starhawk (1987) *Truth or Dare: Encounters with Power, Authority and Mystery.* New York, NY: Harper Collins.

Stevenson, L. (1998) 'Rites and Responsibility for Resuscitation in Heart Failure: Tread Gently on the Thin Places.' *Circulation 98*, 7, 619–22.

Stoneking, C.B. (2003) 'Modernity: The Social Construction of Aging.' In S. Hauerwas, C.B. Stoneking, K.G. Meador and D. Cloutier (eds) *Growing Old in Christ.* Grand Rapids, MI: Eerdmans.

Sutcliffe, D. (1988) *Working with Alzheimer's Disease.* Eastbourne: Ullswater Publications.

Swinton, J. (2000a) *Resurrecting the Person: Friendship and the Care of People with Severe Mental Health Problems.* Nashville, TN: Abingdon Press.

Swinton, J. (2000b) *From Bedlam to Shalom: Towards a Practical Theology of Human Nature, Interpersonal Relationships and Mental Health Care.* New York, NY: Peter Lang.

Swinton, J. (2001) *Spirituality and Mental Health Care: Rediscovering a 'Forgotten' Dimension.* London: Jessica Kingsley Publishers.

Swinton, J. (ed.) (2004) *Critical Reflections on Stanley Hauerwas' Theology of Disability: Disabling Society, Enabling Theology.* New York, NY: Haworth Pastoral Press.

Swinton, J. and Mowat, H. (2006) *Practical Theology and Qualitative Research.* London: SCM Press.

Thomas, D. (1971) 'Do Not Go Gentle Into That Good Night.' In *Dylan Thomas: The Poems.* London: Dent and Sons.

Thomsen, M. (2004) 'Reflections on the Priority of Belonging.' *Currents in Theology and Mission 31*, 4, 316–21.

Touhy, T.A. (2001) 'Nurturing Hope and Spirituality in the Nursing Home.' *Holistic Nursing Practice 15*, 4, 45–56.

Treanor, C. (2006) Unpublished song.

Treanor, C. and Vincent, P. (2006) 'Something about Ann.' In P. Mowbray (ed.) *We Have a Story*, Australian Catholic Bishops Conference. Used with permission.

Trevitt, C. and MacKinlay, E. (2006) 'I Am Just an Ordinary Person …': Spiritual Reminiscence in Older People with Memory Loss.' *Journal of Religion, Spirituality and Aging 18*, 2/3, 77–89.

Trewin, D. (2004) *Suicides: Recent Trends, Australia (1993–2003)*. Canberra: Australian Bureau of Statistics.

Turner, V. (1969) *The Ritual Process*. London: Routledge and Kegan Paul.

Uekermann, J, Channon, S. and Daum, I. (2006) 'Humor Processing, Mentalizing, and Executive Function in Normal Aging.' *Journal of the International Neuropsychological Society 12*, 184–91.

Vanier, J. (2004) 'Response: The Need of Strangers.' In J. Swinton (ed.) *Critical Reflections on Stanley Hauerwas' Theology of Disability*. New York, NY: Haworth Press, 27–30.

Volf, M. (1996) *Exclusion and Embrace: A Theological Exploration of Identity, Otherness and Reconciliation*. Nashville: Abingdon.

Walker, A. (1984) *In Search of Our Mothers' Gardens: Womanist Prose*. London: The Women's Press.

Ward, H. and Wild, J. (1995) *Human Rites: Worship Resources for an Age of Change*. London: Mowbray.

Weil, S. (1974) *Gateway to God*, trans. D. Raper. London: Fontana.

Welch, S. (1990) *A Feminist Ethic of Risk*. Minneapolis, MN: Fortress.

Wendell, S. (1989) 'Towards a Feminist Theory of Disability.' *Hypatia 4*, 2, 104–24.

Wenham, G.J. (1994) *Genesis 16–50*, vol. 2, Word Biblical Commentary. Milton Keynes: Word Publishing.

Westermann, C. (1985) *Genesis 12–36*, trans. J.J. Scullion. London: SPCK.

Whitehead, E. and Whitehead, J. (1995) *Seasons of Strength: New Visions of Adult Christian Maturing*. Winona, MN: St Mary's Press.

Wicks, R., and Rodgerson, T. (1998) *Companions in Hope*. New York, NY: Paulist.

Williams, B. (1998) *Naked Before God*. Harrisburg, PA: Morehouse Publishing.

Williams, J. (1988) 'Mothers, Chaos and Prayer.' In M. Furlong (ed.) *Mirror to the Church: Reflections on Sexism*. London: SPCK.

Williams, P. (2000) *Buddhist Thought: A Complete Introduction to the Indian Tradition* London and New York, NY: Routledge.

Willimon, W. (1979) *Worship as Pastoral Care*. Nashville, TN: Abingdon.

Winnicott, D.W. (1971) *Playing and Reality*. London: Routledge.

Winnicott, D.W. (1986) *Home is Where We Start From: Essays by a Psychoanalyst*. London: Routledge.

Winterson, J. (1995) *Art Objects: Essays on Ecstasy and Effrontery*. London: Vintage.

Woods, B. (2005) 'Dementia.' In M.L. Johnson, V.L. Bengtson, P.G. Coleman and T.B.L. Kirkwood (eds) *The Cambridge Handbook of Age and Ageing.* Cambridge: Cambridge University Press, 252–60.

Wurm, A. (1996) 'Women and the Anglican Church.' In D. Hodge (ed.) *The Fall Upwards: Spirituality in the Lives of Lesbian Women and Gay Men.* Casuarina, NT: Little Gem.

Yesavage, J.A., Brink, T.L., Rose, T.L., Lum, O. *et al.* (1983) 'Development and Validation of a Geriatric Depression Screening Scale: A Preliminary Report.' *Journal of Psychiatric Research 17,* 37–49.

Ziettlow, J. (2004) *The Stages of Faith Development.* Chicago, IL: Evangelical Lutheran Church in America.

Zimmerman, S. (1991) 'Ageing in L'Arche.' *Letters of L'Arche 68,* 2, 5–8.

Contributors

Rev. Dr Matthew Anstey, a deacon in the Anglican Church, is an Australian Research Council Postdoctoral Fellow (2006–2009) at Charles Sturt University School of Theology, conducting research in the area of Biblical Hebrew linguistics, and lecturing in Old Testament. In addition to Hebrew, Matthew has a particular interest in Old Testament interpretation and homiletics, and the contribution of the Old Testament to theology, pastoral care, spirituality, and aesthetics.

Mrs Christine Bryden was diagnosed with dementia in 1995. As a 46-year-old single mother of three girls, Christine then wrote two books *Who Will I Be When I Die* and *Dancing with Dementia*. She become a national and international advocate for people with dementia, and was the first person with dementia to be elected to the Board of Alzheimer's Disease International in 2003. Christine has spoken at major Alzheimer's and related conferences in Australia (including ACSA National Conference Hobart 2004) and overseas. Copies of her talks are available from her website, www.christinebryden.com.

Much of **Dagmar Ceramidas'** three decades as an occupational therapist has been in mental health, particularly depression across the lifespan. She is the Chair of the International Advisory Group on Mental Health for her profession; is a Board Member of Suicide Prevention Australia, and has served as a Board Member on the Mental Health Council of Australia. Dagmar lectures and researches with the Centre for Ageing and Pastoral Studies, Charles Sturt University. The conference paper presentation was supported by a grant from The Centre for Public and Contextual Theology (PACT) at Charles Sturt University.

Eileen Glass AM has been a member of L'Arche for more than thirty years. For ten years she lived in community households with people with intellectual disabilities, in Canada and Australia. During the 1990s she coordinated L'Arche communities in Asia and the western Pacific, working with people in a variety of cultural and religious settings. Currently she works as a Spiritual Director, offering retreats and formation within L'Arche and beyond. Of particular interest to her are retreats for people with intellectual disability.

Rev. Malcolm Goldsmith was ordained in 1962. After a varied ministry in which he was a parish priest, a university chaplain, a chaplain to a hospice, a Bishop's adviser on Industry, and a research fellow in dementia studies he retired in 2002. His book *Hearing the Voice of People with Dementia* was shortlisted for the Seebohm Prize, 'for the book which best promotes the well-being and understanding of older people'. He has also published *In a Strange Land: People with Dementia and the Local Church*. In his retirement he writes, paints and delights in his grandchildren.

Dr Lorna Hallahan is a social worker and theologian with over twenty years' experience of working for social justice and decency, particularly in the disability movement. A lecturer in social work at Flinders University, Lorna is very wary of 'gooey' spirituality and is committed to keeping spirit and action for social justice and decency securely linked.

Lorna, who has a mobility impairment, lives in the Adelaide foothills with her partner, a legal aid lawyer, their two sons and a fine flock of bantam hens.

Associate Professor Rosalie Hudson is a consultant/educator in aged care, palliative care and pastoral care. She is an honorary senior fellow in the School of Nursing, the University of Melbourne; she teaches in undergraduate and postgraduate nursing programmes and is a contracted educator with Alzheimer's Victoria. She has twelve years' experience as director of nursing of an aged care facility. She has published widely on many aspects of aged care in both nursing and theological journals. Her fourth co-authored book, *Palliative Care and Aged Care*, was published in 2007. Rosalie is a regular speaker at conferences both nationally and internationally.

Rev. Dr Elizabeth MacKinlay AM is a registered nurse and a priest in the Anglican Church of Australia and the Director of the Centre for Ageing and Pastoral Studies at St Mark's National Theological Centre, Canberra. She is Associate Professor, School of Theology, Charles Sturt University, a Principal Researcher in the Designated Research Centre for Public and Contextual Theology (PACT), CSU, and Chair of the ACT Ministerial Advisory Council on Ageing.

Rev. Dr Laurence McNamara is Senior Lecturer in Christian Ethics at the Catholic Theological College in the Adelaide College of Divinity and the School of Theology, Flinders University, South Australia. He is a Roman Catholic priest. Following graduate studies in Rome and Oxford he obtained his PhD at the University of Adelaide. His research interests are focused on the theological, ethical, spiritual and pastoral care aspects of human ageing. He has also developed a nationally recognized Diploma of Ageing and Pastoral Care for pastoral care workers in residential and community aged care settings.

Dr Carmen Moran has researched, taught and practised as a psychologist in a variety of areas related to health and well-being, most recently in the School of Social Sciences and International Relations at the University of New South Wales. Her research looks at both negative and positive aspects of coping under stress, especially in extreme environments, such as emergency work and war. In recent years, this research has focused on humour and on spirituality, and their independent and combined relationships to stress, coping, and well-being. She has published in these areas, and presented her work at local and international conferences.

Rev. Dr Christopher Newell AM is Associate Professor in Medical Ethics in the School of Medicine, University of Tasmania and Canon Theologian at St David's Cathedral, Hobart. He is also an Adjunct Lecturer in theological ethics at Trinity College Theological School in Melbourne. Current board memberships include the Australian National Health and Medical Research Council and the Australian Commission for Safety and Quality in Health Care. Recent books include *Digital Disability* (2003), *From Out Back to Out Front: Voices in Spirituality and Disability from the Land Down Under* (2004), *Disability in Australia* (2005) and *Disability in Education* (2005).

Rev. Dr Alan Niven teaches at Melbourne College of Divinity and is Vice-Principal/ Lecturer in Pastoral and Family Studies at the Churches of Christ Theological College (CCTC), Mulgrave, Victoria. His interest in practical theology and his consequent teaching areas have developed through parish ministry, marriage and family education, and pastoral counselling. As a Board Member of Churches of Christ Community Care (Victoria) he also oversees a new CCTC ministry formation programme for Aged Care Intern-Chaplains at a number of facilities in Melbourne.

Rev. Dr Ruwan Palapathwala lectures in the fields of Pastoral Theology and Religion and Culture at Trinity College, the University of Melbourne and in Asian Religions in the United Faculty of Theology of the Melbourne College of Divinity. His specializations are in the religions of South and Southeast Asia, the intertextuality of the Holy Books and Christian theology. He is a priest in the Anglican Archdiocese of Melbourne and the Director of the Centre for Social Inquiry, Religion and Interfaith Dialogue (Melbourne).

Kirstin Robertson-Gillam has been a Music Therapist, Registered Nurse and Counsellor for 26 years with experience in aged care, palliative care, mental health and disabilities. She gives casual lectures in music therapy at both university-based courses in Sydney, Australia. She created the *Spirited Living Program*® which utilizes imagery, music and meditation for people of all ages to motivate and improve health. Kirstin is currently doing Masters Honours Research at the University of

Western Sydney, focused on the effectiveness of vocal improvisation and choir work with a counselling orientation to reduce depression in people with dementia.

Rev. Prof. John Swinton holds the chair in Practical Theology and Pastoral Care at the University of Aberdeen, Scotland, United Kingdom. For 16 years he practised as a registered nurse specializing in psychiatry and learning disabilities and for a number of years he was a mental health chaplain. He is director of the Centre for Spirituality, Health and Disability (www.abdn.ac.uk/cshad). His books include *Spirituality and Mental Health Care: Rediscovering a 'Forgotten' Dimension* (Jessica Kingsley Publishers 2001) and *Raging with Compassion: Pastoral Responses to the Problem of Evil* (Eerdmans 2007).

Subject Index

Author Index

French, S. 41
Frey, B. 185, 187, 195, 198
Friedman, D. 222, 223
Fulghum, R. 217, 220, 228, 232

Gardner, W. L. 173, 176
Gennep, A. van 219, 226
George, L. 183
George, L. K. 164
Gerkin, C. V. 107, 117
Gerster, R. 204
Gibson, F. 192, 195
Gibson, G. 218
Gibson, R. 218
Glaser, B. G. 164
Glass, E. 10, 17, 49, 237
Goggin, G. 73, 74, 78
Goldberg, M. 108
Goldsmith, M. 10, 17, 18, 84, 122, 235
Goulart, J. 221

Habermas, J. 229
Haight, B. K. 106
Hales, C. 161
Hall, K. 67, 68, 70
Hallahan, R. 13, 95
Halpern, A. 190
Hauerwas, S. 14–15, 19, 83, 106, 108
Herr, S. 73–4
Hickie, I. B. 175
Hill, R. D. 175
Hudson, R. 10, 19, 85, 236
Huggett, J. 121
Hughes, D. 183
Hughes, J. C. 16, 235, 236
Hutchison, M. 32
Hybels, C. F. 176

Idler, E. L. 164
Imber-Black, E. 220, 224, 225, 227
Iozzio, M. J. 33, 34
Isaiah, D. 184

Jackson, J. P. 174, 176
Jamieson, D. 107
Jayatilake, K. N. 162

Jeremiah, M. 125
Jewell, A. 106
Johnson, J. 189
Johnston, M. 208
Jones, L. G. 108
Jones, T. P. 166
Jorm, A. F. 163
Joyner, R. 173

Kahn, R. 11
Kaldor, P. 164
Kalupahana, D. J. 162
Kaplan, H. I. 163, 171, 173, 175, 177
Kass, L. R. 109, 112
Katz, S. 158
Kaut, K. 185
Kazniak, A. 183
Kehn, D. J. 164
Kelly, A. 100
Kelly, K. 65
Kenyon, G. M. 19, 53, 106
Killick, J. 84, 186
Kimble, M. A. 18, 52, 89
Kitwood, T. 14, 26–8, 29, 33, 52, 82, 235
Kivnick, H. 192
Knox, I. S. 106
Koder, S. 164
Koenig, H. G. 106, 107, 164, 184, 185, 234
Kopelman, L. M. 43
Krause, N. M. 164
Kuchibhatia, M. 184
Kugel, J. L. 109

L'Arche Ontario 65
LaCugna, C. 85
Laffin, J. 208
Lake-Smith, T. 166
Lambert, E. 208
Lapsley, J. 148
Larson 185
Laugesen, A. 208
Lear, J. 147
Lee, J. 97
Lefcourt, H. 203, 209, 215
Levin, J. S. 164
Lewis, A. 87
Lewis, J. 219

Lewis, M. 183
Llewellyn-Jones, R. 183
Looi, J. 163
Loois, J. C. L. 209
Lopez, S. 185
Louw, S. J. 16, 235
Lunsford, D. A. 158
Luszcz, M. 184

MacIntyre, A. 41, 92
MacKinlay, E. 10, 14, 17, 51, 52, 53, 86, 106, 107, 183, 185, 211, 214, 215, 219, 222, 223, 234, 235
Macleod, D. 166
Maddox, G. L. 39, 41
Magalhães, J. P. 146
Marshall, B. 158
Martin, R. A. 203
Massam, M. 201, 204, 206, 208
Mauritzen, J. 184–5
May, W. F. 37, 38
McBee, L. 188
McCullough, M. 185
McFadden, S. H. 164, 211
McHugh, P. 182
McKee, K. J. 210
McNamara, L. 10, 12, 15, 19, 235
McSherry, W. 220, 222, 234
Meador, K. G. 176
Meares, R. 108
Meilaender, G. 84
Mitchell, J. 231
Moberg, D. O. 106, 164
Modell, S. M. 107
Moltmann, J. 29, 221, 222, 223, 225–6
Moody, H. 98
Moody, H. R. 234
Moore, H, 96
Moran, C. 10, 20, 201, 204, 205, 206, 208, 209
Morgan, R. L. 106
Moriarty, G. 169
Morley, J. 221